Alkaline Diet Cookbook for Beginners

2 Books in 1 | Dr. Lewis's Meal Plan Project | 200 Child-Friendly Recipes to Make Your Transformation Path Tastier and More Effective (Premium Edition)

By Grace Lewis

Copyright © 2021 Grace Lewis

All rights reserved.

ISBN: 978-1-80311-088-2 (Paperback Color)

ISBN: 978-1-80311-089-9 (Hardcover Color)

Table of Contents

Alkaline Diet Cookbook for Men

Alkaline Diet Cookbook on a Budget

Alkaline Diet Cookbook for Men

Dr. Lewis's Meal Plan Project| 100 Specific Recipes to Keep Body Acids Under Control| Find the Well-Being You've Always Wished for Thanks to an Effective and Easy-To-Follow Path.

By Grace Lewis

Chapter 1 - Introduction

This book was written for all men who have made the choice to embark on a journey of transforming their lives.

The alkaline diet is the simplest and most effective way to begin a long-term journey of transformation.

Below we will answer some questions that people usually ask me during private sessions

What is an alkaline diet?

The premise of an alkaline diet is this: replace acidic foods with alkaline foods and your health will improve. Why would this work, you may ask? The theory is that by regulating your body's pH level (pH is a scientific scale on which acids and bases are measured), you can lose weight and avoid chronic diseases such as cancer and heart disease. pH is measured on a scale of 1 to 14; below seven are the most acidic foods, such as vinegar, animal fats and dairy products. Above seven are the alkaline foods, which mostly include healthy, plant-based foods. When we digest a food, we are left with residual ash, which can be acidic or alkaline. Therefore, an alkaline diet is sometimes called an alkaline ash diet. Proponents of the alkaline diet say that acidic ash can be dangerous to your health.

Is an alkaline diet healthy?

Processed meats are high on cancer doctors' list of foods never to eat, and they are also condemned in the alkaline diet because of their high acidity. "An alkaline diet is a diet that seeks to balance the body's pH levels by increasing the consumption of alkalizing foods such as fruits and vegetables and reducing/eliminating most acidifying foods such as processed meats and refined grains," explains Josh Axe, DNM, author of Eat Dirt and co-founder of Ancient Nutrition.

Can an alkaline diet reduce the risk of cancer?

Many anti-cancer foods are also alkaline diet foods, but there is currently no evidence for or against the role of alkaline diets in cancer prevention. However, plant-based diets are thought to help reduce the risk of cancer and are even recommended for cancer survivors, according to the American Institute for Cancer Research. New research from the University of Alabama at Birmingham suggests that a plant-based diet may make it easier to treat one of the deadliest forms of breast cancer. Although the evidence is somewhat contradictory: some chemotherapy drugs kill more cancer cells in an alkaline environment, while others work better in an acidic environment, according to a review in the Journal of Environmental Public Health. It's worth discussing this with your doctor if you are being treated for cancer.

At the end of the manual, you'll find my personal method designed for a male audience to get you started on the recipes in this book right away.

Enjoy!

Grace

Alkaline Diet
Breakfast
Recipes

1) Blueberry Muffins

Preparation time: 1 hour

Cooking time:

Servings: 3

Ingredients:

- ✓ 1/2 cup of Blueberries
- ✓ 3/4 cup of Teff Flour
- ✓ 3/4 cup of Spelt Flour
- ✓ 1/3 cup of Agave Syrup

Directions:

- ❖ Preheat our oven to 365 degrees Fahrenheit.
- ❖ Grate or line up 6 standard muffin cups.
- ❖ Add the yeast, sifted flour, sifted mashed potato, nut milk, peanut butter, and agave juice to a large bowl.

Ingredients:

- ✓ 1/2 teaspoon of Pure Sea Salt
- ✓ 1 cup of Coconut Milk
- ✓ 1/4 cup Sea Moss Gel seed oil (optional, check information)

- ❖ Put them in order for a while.
- ❖ Add the blueberries to the mixture and mix well.
- ❖ Divide muffin batter among 6 muffin cups.
- ❖ Bake for 30 minutes until golden brown.
- ❖ Experiment and enjoy our Blueberry Muffins!

Helpful Hints:

2) Banana Strawberry Ice Crem

Preparation time:

Cooking time: 4 Hours

Servings: 5

Ingredients:

- ✓ 1 cup of Strawberry*.
- ✓ 5 quartered Baby Bananas*.
- ✓ 1/2 Avocado, chopped

Directions:

- ❖ Put all the ingredients in and let them dry well.
- ❖ Taste. If so, add more milk or agave syrup if you want it to be more full-bodied.

Ingredients:

- ✓ 1 tablespoon of Agave syrup
- ✓ 1/4 cup of walnut milk Homemade

- ❖ Place in a container with a lid and let mash for at least 5-6 hours.
- ❖ Serve and enjoy your Bana Strawberry Ice creamy!

Helpful hints: If you don't fresh berries or banas, you can use frozen ones. You can use as much fruit as you want, but be sure to use only fresh fruit. The fat in the Avocado helps make a creamier consistency. If you don't have homemade nut milk, you can substitute it with homemade sheep's milk.

3) Chocolate cream Homemade Whipped

Preparation time: 10 Minutes.

Cooking time:

Servings: 1 cup

Ingredients:

✓ *1 cup of Aquafaba*

Directions:

- ❖ Add Agave Syrup and Aquafaba into a bowl.
- ❖ Mix to the height speed about 5 minutes with a mixer stand
  - o 10 to 15 minutes with a mixer hand.

Ingredients:

- ✓ 1/4 cup of Agave Syrup

- ❖ Serve and enjoy our Homemade Whipped Cream!

Helpful Hints: Keep in the refrigerator if not using immediately. The whipped cream will become Aquafaba consistency eventually, until set.

4) "Chocolate" Pudding.

Preparation time: **Cooking time:** 20 Minutes.   **Servings: 4**

Ingredients:

- ✓ 1 to 2 cups of Black Sapote
- ✓ 1/4 cup agave syrup
- ✓ 1/2 cup of soaked Brazil Nuts (overnight or at least 3 hours)

Directions:

- ❖ Cut 1 or 2 cups of Black Sapote in half.
- ❖ Remove all the seeds. You should have 1 cup ou full of fruit de-seded.

Ingredients:

- ✓ 1 tablespoon of hemp seeds
- ✓ 1/2 cup of Spring Water

- ❖ Place all ingredients in a blender and blend until smooth.
- ❖ Serve and enjoy our chocolate pudding!

Helpful Hints: Store in the refrigerator when not in use. You can use it with our Homemade whipped crust.

5) Walnut muffins

Preparation time: **Cooking time:** 1 hour   **Servings: 6**

Ingredients:

- ✓ Dry ingredients:
- ✓ 1 1/2 cups of Spell or Teff Flour
- ✓ 1/2 teaspoon of Pure Sea Salt
- ✓ 3/4 cup of Date Syrup
- ✓ What's the problem?
- ✓ 2 medium pureed Burro Banas

Directions:

- ❖ Preheat the oven to 400 degrees.
- ❖ Take a muffin tray and grease 12 cups or line with cupcake liners.
- ❖ Place all dry ingredients in a large bowl and mix well.
- ❖ Add all ingredients to a larger bowl and mix with the Bin Laden. 5. Mix the ingredients from the two bowls into one container. Be careful not to over mix.

Ingredients:

- ✓ ¼ cup of ground soybean oil
- ✓ ¾ cup of Homemade Walnut Milk *
- ✓ 1 tablespoon of Key Lime Juice
- ✓ Ingredients for filling:
- ✓ ½ cup of chopped Walnuts (plus extra for decorating)
- ✓ 1 banana burrita
- ❖ Add the filling ingredients and fry.
- ❖ Place our batter in the 12 muffin cups and fill them with a knob of butter.
- ❖ Bake 22 to 26 mnutes until golden brown.
- ❖ Allow to cool for 10 minutes.
- ❖ Serve and enjoy your Bana Nut Muffins!

6) Banana and almond smoothie

Preparation time: 10 minutes   **Cooking time:** 0 minutes   **Servings: 2**

Ingredients:

- ✓ 2 large frozen bananas, peeled and sliced
- ✓ 1 tablespoon chopped almonds

Directions:

- ❖ Place all ingredients in a high speed blender and pulse until smooth and creamy.

Ingredients:

- ✓ 1 teaspoon of organic vanilla extract
- ✓ 2 cups of cooled unsweetened almond milk

- ❖ Pour smoothie into two serving glasses and serve immediately

7) _Strawberry and Beet Smoothie_

Preparation time: 10 minutes   **Cooking time**: 0 minutes   **Servings: 2**

Ingredients:

- ✓ 2 cups frozen strawberries, hulled
- ✓ 2/3 cup frozen beets, cut, peeled and chopped
- ✓ 1 teaspoon of fresh ginger root, peeled and grated

Directions:

- ❖ Place all ingredients in a high speed blender and pulse until smooth and creamy.

Ingredients:

- ✓ 1 teaspoon fresh turmeric root, peeled and grated
- ✓ ½ cup of fresh orange juice
- ✓ 1 cup unsweetened almond milk

- ❖ Pour smoothie into two serving glasses and serve immediately

8) _Raspberry and tofu smoothie_

Preparation time: 10 minutes   **Cooking time:**   **Servings: 2**

Ingredients:

- ✓ 1½ cups of fresh raspberries
- ✓ 6 ounces of firm silken tofu, drained, pressed and chopped
- ✓ 1 teaspoon of stevia powder

Directions:

- ❖ Place all ingredients in a high speed blender and pulse until smooth and creamy.

Ingredients:

- ✓ 1/8 teaspoon of organic vanilla extract
- ✓ 1½ cups unsweetened almond milk
- ✓ ¼ cup ice cubes, crushed

- ❖ Pour smoothie into two serving glasses and serve immediately

9) _Mango and lemon smoothie_

Preparation time: 10 minutes   **Cooking time:**   **Servings: 2**

Ingredients:

- ✓ 2 cups frozen mango, peeled, pitted and chopped
- ✓ ¼ cup almond butter
- ✓ pinch of ground turmeric

Directions:

- ❖ Place all ingredients in a high speed blender and pulse until smooth and creamy.

Ingredients:

- ✓ 2 tablespoons fresh lemon juice
- ✓ 1¼ cup unsweetened almond milk
- ✓ ¼ cup ice cubes, crushed

- ❖ Pour smoothie into two serving glasses and serve immediately

10) Papaya and banana smoothie

Preparation time: 10 minutes   **Cooking time:**   **Servings: 2**

Ingredients:
- ½ of a medium papaya, peeled and coarsely chopped
- 1 large banana, peeled and sliced
- 2 tablespoons of agave nectar
- ¼ teaspoon ground turmeric

Directions:
- Place all ingredients in a high speed blender and pulse until smooth and creamy.

Ingredients:
- 1 tablespoon fresh lime juice
- 1½ cups unsweetened almond milk
- ½ cup ice cubes, crushed

- Pour smoothie into two serving glasses and serve immediately

11) Orange and Oat Smoothie

Preparation time: 10 minutes   **Cooking time:**   **Servings: 2**

Ingredients:
- 2/3 cups rolled oats
- 2 oranges, peeled, with seeds and cut into pieces
- 2 large bananas, peeled and sliced

Directions:
- Place all ingredients in a high speed blender and pulse until smooth and creamy.

Ingredients:
- 1½ cups unsweetened almond milk
- ½ cup ice cubes, crushed

- Pour smoothie into two serving glasses and serve immediately

12) Pineapple and Kale Smoothie

Preparation time: 10 minutes   **Cooking time:**   **Servings: 2**

Ingredients:
- 1½ cups fresh cabbage, hard ribs removed and chopped
- 1 large frozen banana, peeled and sliced
- ½ cup fresh pineapple, peeled and cut into pieces

Directions:
- Place all ingredients in a high speed blender and pulse until smooth and creamy.

Ingredients:
- ½ cup of fresh orange juice
- 1 cup unsweetened coconut milk
- ½ cup ice cubes, crushed
- Pour smoothie into two serving glasses and serve immediately

13) Pumpkin and Banana Smoothie

Preparation time: 10 minutes   **Cooking time:**   **Servings: 2**

Ingredients:
- 1 cup homemade pumpkin puree
- 1 large banana, peeled and sliced
- 1 tablespoon maple syrup
- 1 teaspoon ground flax seeds

Directions:
- Place all ingredients in a high speed blender and pulse until smooth and creamy.

Ingredients:
- ¼ teaspoon of cinnamon powder
- 1/8 teaspoon ground ginger
- 1½ cups unsweetened almond milk
- ¼ cup ice cubes, crushed
- Pour smoothie into two serving glasses and serve immediately

14) *Cabbage and avocado smoothie*

Preparation time: 10 minutes   **Cooking time**:   **Servings: 2**

Ingredients:
- ✓ 2 cups fresh cabbage, hard ribs removed and chopped
- ✓ ½ of a medium avocado, peeled, pitted and chopped
- ✓ ½ inch pieces of fresh ginger root, peeled and chopped

Directions:
- ❖ Place all ingredients in a high speed blender and pulse until smooth and creamy.

Ingredients:
- ✓ ½ inch pieces of fresh turmeric root, peeled and chopped
- ✓ 1½ cups unsweetened coconut milk
- ✓ ¼ cup ice cubes, crushed
- ❖ Pour smoothie into two serving glasses and serve immediately

15) *Cucumber and Herb Smoothie*

Preparation time: 10 minutes   **Cooking time**:   **Servings: 2**

Ingredients:
- ✓ 2 cups fresh mixed vegetables (cabbage, beets), chopped and shredded
- ✓ 1 small cucumber, peeled and chopped
- ✓ ½ cup of lettuce, torn
- ✓ ¼ cup fresh parsley leaves
- ✓ ¼ cup fresh mint leaves

Directions:
- ❖ Place all ingredients in a high speed blender and pulse until smooth and creamy.

Ingredients:
- ✓ 2-3 drops of liquid stevia
- ✓ 1 teaspoon fresh lemon juice
- ✓ 1½ cups of alkaline water
- ✓ ¼ cup ice cubes, crushed

16) *Hemp seed and carrot muffins*

Pour smoothie into two serving glasses and serve immediately

Preparation time: 20-25 minutes   **Cooking time**:   **Servings: 12**

Ingredients:
- ✓ Cashew butter, 6 tablespoons
- ✓ Shredded Carrot,
- ✓ Unrefined whole cane sugar, .5 c.
- ✓ Almond milk, 1 c.
- ✓ Oatmeal, 2 c.
- ✓ Ground flaxseed, 1 tablespoon

Directions:
- ❖ Start by setting your oven to 350.
- ❖ Whisk the flax seeds and water together to make the flax egg.
- ❖ Pour everything into a larger bowl and then combine the salt, vanilla powder, baking powder, kale, hemp seeds, cashew butter, carrot, sugar, almond milk and oatmeal.

Ingredients:
- ✓ Water, 3 tablespoons
- ✓ Pinch of sea salt
- ✓ Powdered vanilla bean, one pinch
- ✓ Baking powder, 1 tablespoon
- ✓ Chopped cabbage, 1 tablespoon
- ✓ Hemp seeds, 2 tablespoons
- ❖ Mix everything together until well combined.
- ❖ Grease a 12-cup muffin pan and divide the batter between the cups. Bake for 20-25 minutes and enjoy.

17) Chia seed and strawberry parfait

Preparation time: **Cooking time:** **Servings: 2**

Ingredients:

- ✓ Strawberry mixture -
- ✓ Brown rice syrup, 1-2 teaspoons
- ✓ Chia seeds, 1 teaspoon
- ✓ Diced strawberries, 1 c.
- ✓ Oat Blend -

Directions:

- ❖ To make the strawberry mixture, mix together the brown rice syrup, chia seeds and strawberries in a small bowl until well blended.
- ❖ In a separate bowl, mix together the vanilla bean powder, brown rice syrup, coconut milk and oats until well blended.

Ingredients:

- ✓ Quick rolled oats, 1 c.
- ✓ Powdered vanilla bean, one pinch
- ✓ Brown rice syrup, 1 tablespoon
- ✓ Coconut milk, 1 c.

- ❖ Place one part of the oats in the base of two jars. Cover with some of the strawberry mixture. Repeat with the remaining ingredients.
- ❖ Put a lid on the jars and let them sit in the fridge overnight.
- ❖ The next morning, discover and enjoy.

18) Pecan Pancakes

Preparation time: **Cooking time:** **Servings: 5**

Ingredients:

- ✓ Chopped pecans, .25 c.
- ✓ Nutmeg, .25 tsp
- ✓ Cinnamon, 0.5 teaspoons
- ✓ Vanilla, 1 teaspoon
- ✓ Melted butter, 2 tablespoons
- ✓ Unsweetened soy milk, .75 c.

Directions:

- ❖ Place the salt, sugar substitute, baking powder and almond flour in a bowl and mix well.
- ❖ In another bowl, place the vanilla, soy milk, butter and eggs. Stir well to incorporate everything.
- ❖ Place the egg mixture into the dry contents and mix well until well blended.
- ❖ Add the nutmeg, pecans and cinnamon. Stir for five minutes.

Ingredients:

- ✓ Eggs, 2
- ✓ Salt, .25 tsp
- ✓ Baking powder, .25 tsp
- ✓ Granular sugar substitute, 1 tablespoon
- ✓ Almond flour, .75 c.
- ✓ Olive oil - cooking spray
- ❖ Place a 12-inch skillet over medium heat and sprinkle with cooking spray.
- ❖ Pour one tablespoon of batter into the preheated pan and spread into a four-inch circle.
- ❖ Pour three more spoonfuls into the pan and cook until bubbles have formed at the edges of the pancakes and the bottom is golden brown.
- ❖ Turn each one over and cook an additional two minutes.
- ❖ Repeat the process until all the batter has been used.
- ❖ Serve with a syrup of your choice.

19) Quinoa Breakfast

Preparation time: **Cooking time:** **Servings: 4**

Ingredients:

- ✓ Maple syrup, 3 tablespoons
- ✓ 2 inch cinnamon stick
- ✓ Water, 2 c.
- ✓ Quinoa, 1 c.
- ✓ Optional Condiments:
- ✓ Yogurt
- ✓ Chopped cashews, 2 tablespoons

Directions:

- ❖ Place the quinoa in a colander and rinse under cold running water. Make sure there are no stones or anything else.
- ❖ Pour the water into a saucepan, add the quinoa and place the saucepan over medium heat. Bring to a boil.

Ingredients:

- ✓ Whipped coconut cream, 3 tablespoons
- ✓ Lime juice, 1 teaspoon
- ✓ Nutmeg, .25 tsp
- ✓ Raisins, 2 tablespoons
- ✓ Strawberries, .5 c.
- ✓ Raspberries, .5 c.
- ✓ Blueberries, .5 c.
- ❖ Add the cinnamon stick, put a lid on the saucepan, lower the hot temperature, even, simmer gently fifteen minutes until the water is engulfed.
- ❖ Remove from hot temperature and stir with a fork. Add maple syrup and one of the toppings listed above.

20) Oatmeal

Preparation time:　　　　**Cooking time:**　　　　**Servings: 4**

Ingredients:

- ✓　Halls
- ✓　Steel cut oats, 1.25 c.
- ✓　Water, 3.75 c.
- ✓　Optional Condiments:
- ✓　Nuts
- ✓　Dried fruits
- ✓　Sliced banana
- ✓　Mango cubes

Ingredients:

- ✓　Mixed berries
- ✓　Garam masala, 1 teaspoon
- ✓　Lemon pepper, .25 tsp
- ✓　Nutmeg, .25 tsp
- ✓　Cinnamon, 1 teaspoon

Directions:

- ❖　Place a saucepan on medium and add the water. Allow the water to boil.
- ❖　Pour in the oats with a pinch of salt and lower the heat to a simmer.

- ❖　Let simmer 25 minutes, stirring constantly.
- ❖　Once all the water has been absorbed, add one of the seasonings listed above if you want to add some flavor. If you want it creamier, add a tablespoon of coconut milk.

21) Sweet spinach salad

Preparation time: **Cooking time:**   **Portions:**

Ingredients:

- ✓ Crushed black pepper (1 teaspoon)
- ✓ Salt (1 teaspoon)
- ✓ Nutmeg (1 teaspoon)
- ✓ Cinnamon (1 teaspoon)
- ✓ Chopped spinach (4 c.)
- ✓ Chopped parsley (2 tablespoons)

Directions:

- ❖ To start this recipe, bring out a large bowl and combine all the ingredients together.

Ingredients:

- ✓ Chopped walnuts (.25 c.)
- ✓ Raisins (.25 c.)
- ✓ Sliced apple (.5 c.)
- ✓ Yogurt (.5 c.)
- ✓ Lime juice (1 tablespoon)
- ✓ Shredded carrots (.75 c.)
- ❖ Place the bowl in the refrigerator to chill for about ten minutes before serving.

22) Steamed green bowl

Preparation time: **Cooking time:**   **Portions:**

Ingredients:

- ✓ Chopped coriander (2 tablespoons)
- ✓ Salt (1 teaspoon)
- ✓ Sliced green onions (2)
- ✓ Ground cashews (1 c.)
- ✓ Coconut milk (2 c.)
- ✓ Green peas (.5 c.)
- ✓ Sliced zucchini (1)

Directions:

- ❖ Heat some coconut oil in a pan and when hot, add the ginger, turmeric, garlic and onion.
- ❖ After five minutes of cooking, add the coconut milk, peas, zucchini and broccoli to this mixture.

Ingredients:

- ✓ Head of broccoli (1)
- ✓ Grated ginger (1 inch)
- ✓ Turmeric (1 teaspoon)
- ✓ Chopped garlic clove (1)
- ✓ Sliced onion (1)
- ✓ Coconut oil (1 tablespoon)

- ❖ Let the ingredients come to a boil before reducing the heat and simmering for a bit.
- ❖ After another 15 minutes, stir in the cilantro, salt, green onions and cashews before serving.

23) Vegetable and berry salad

Preparation time: **Cooking time:**   **Portions:**

Ingredients:

- ✓ Raspberries (.5 c.)
- ✓ Sliced tangerine (.5)
- ✓ Alfalfa sprouts (1 c.)
- ✓ Shredded red cabbage (.5 head)
- ✓ Lemon juice 1
- ✓ Olive oil (3 tablespoons)
- ✓ Diced cucumber (1)
- ✓ Avocado (1)
- ✓ Sliced shallot (1)

Directions:

- ❖ Take a large bowl and add all the ingredients to it.

Ingredients:

- ✓ Sliced cabbage (4 leaves)
- ✓ Chopped parsley (1 tablespoon)
- ✓ Sliced red bell pepper (.5)
- ✓ Shredded Carrot (1)
- ✓ Crushed almonds (1 tablespoon)
- ✓ Pumpkin seeds (2 tablespoons)

- ❖ Stir well to combine before seasoning the fruits and vegetables with a little lemon juice and a little oil.
- ❖ Serve immediately.

24) Bowl of quinoa and carrots

Preparation time:　　　　**Cooking time:**　　　　**Portions:**

Ingredients:

- ✓ Sliced green onions (2 tablespoons)
- ✓ Black sesame seeds (2 tablespoons)
- ✓ Salt (.25 tsp.)
- ✓ Chopped parsley (3 tablespoons)
- ✓ Lemon juice (.5)
- ✓ Cooked quinoa (2 c.)

Directions:

- ❖ Whisk together the miso and water in a bowl. Then take a frying pan and heat some oil in it.
- ❖ When the oil is hot, add the fennel bulb and carrots and cook for a few minutes, turning when three minutes have passed.

Ingredients:

- ✓ Sliced fennel bulb (1)
- ✓ Carrots, chopped (1 bunch)
- ✓ Olive oil (1 tablespoon)
- ✓ Miso (1 tablespoon)
- ✓ Water (1 c.)

- ❖ Add the water and miso mixture to the pan and reduce the heat to low. Cook with the lid on for a bit. This will take about 20 minutes.
- ❖ While this mixture is cooking, combine together the quinoa with the parsley, lemon juice and salt in a bowl.
- ❖ When the carrots are done, add the mixture on top of the quinoa. Sprinkle the green onions and sesame seeds on top before serving.

25) Grab and Go Wraps

Preparation time:　　　　**Cooking time:**　　　　**Portions:**

Ingredients:

- ✓ Carrot cut into julienne (1)
- ✓ Red bell pepper (.5)
- ✓ Swiss chard greens (4)
- ✓ Salt (.25 tsp.)
- ✓ Diced jalapeno bell pepper (.5)

Directions:

- ❖ Get out your blender or food processor and combine together the salt, jalapeno, shallots, cilantro, lime, avocado and peas. Process to combine, but leave some texture to still be there.

Ingredients:

- ✓ Shallots cut into small cubes (1)
- ✓ Chopped coriander leaves (.25 c.)
- ✓ Lime Juice (1)
- ✓ Avocado (1)
- ✓ Steamed green peas (1 c.)
- ❖ Lay the collards out on the counter and then spread your pea and avocado mixture on top.
- ❖ Add the carrot and bell bell pepper strips before rolling up the collars and secure with a toothpick.
- ❖ Repeat with all ingredients before serving.

26) Walnut Tacos

Preparation time:　　　　**Cooking time:**　　　　**Portions:**

Ingredients:

- ✓ Chopped coriander (1 tablespoon)
- ✓ Nutritional yeast (2 tablespoons)
- ✓ Romaine lettuce leaves (6)
- ✓ Cooked red quinoa (.25 c.)
- ✓ Salt (.25 tsp.)
- ✓ Tamari (1 tablespoon)
- ✓ Coconut amino acids (1 teaspoon)
- ✓ Smoked paprika (.25 tsp.)

Directions:

- ❖ To start this recipe, add the almonds and walnuts to the food processor and puree them.
- ❖ Add the tomatoes and give it a couple of pulses until you have a nice crumbly mixture.
- ❖ From there, add the salt, tamari, coconut aminos, paprika, onion, garlic, chili, cilantro, cumin, and olive oil.

Ingredients:

- ✓ Onion powder (.25 tsp.)
- ✓ Garlic Powder (.25 tsp.)
- ✓ Chilli powder (.25 tsp.)
- ✓ Ground Coriander (1 teaspoon)
- ✓ Ground Cumin (1 teaspoon)
- ✓ Olive oil (2 tablespoons)
- ✓ Chopped dried tomatoes (.25 c.)
- ✓ Chopped raw almonds (.25 c.)
- ✓ Walnuts (.5 c.)
- ❖ It pulses a few more times to be fully combined.
- ❖ Add the tomato and walnut mixture to a bowl and combine with the quinoa.
- ❖ Divide this mixture among the romaine lettuce leaves and top with the cilantro and nutritional yeast before serving.

27) Tex-Mex bowl

Preparation time:

Cooking time:

Portions:

Ingredients:

- ✓ Nutritional yeast (2 tablespoons)
- ✓ Cilantro (2 tablespoons)
- ✓ Sliced avocado (1)
- ✓ Salt (.25 tsp.)
- ✓ Olive oil (.25 c.)
- ✓ Apple Cider Vinegar (.25 c.)
- ✓ Lime juice and zest (1)
- ✓ Lemon juice and zest (1)
- ✓ Squeezed Oranges (2)
- ✓ Chopped garlic cloves (2)
- ✓ Sliced red onion (1)
- ✓ Sliced peppers
- ✓ For the brown rice
- ✓ Hind beans (.5 c.)

Ingredients:

- ✓ Garlic powder (.5 tsp.)
- ✓ Cayenne pepper (.5 tsp.)
- ✓ Paprika (1 teaspoon)
- ✓ Salt (1 teaspoon)
- ✓ Garlic powder (1.5 teaspoons)
- ✓ Chili powder (2 teaspoons)
- ✓ Cooked brown rice (1 c.)
- ✓ Sauce
- ✓ Juice of a lime
- ✓ Salt (.25 tsp.)
- ✓ Diced Cilantro (.25 c.)
- ✓ Diced red onion (.5)
- ✓ Diced Tomatoes (2)

Directions:

- ❖ Pull out a large bowl and combine together the salt, olive oil, vinegar, lime zest and juice, lemon zest and juice, garlic, red onion, and bell bell pepper.
- ❖ Cover and let sit for about five hours to marinate a bit. While the peppers marinate a bit in the refrigerator, it's time to work on the sauce.
- ❖ To make the sauce, add all ingredients to a small bowl and mix well to combine. Cover the bowl and place in the refrigerator.

- ❖ In a medium bowl, add all the ingredients for the brown rice. Mix well and set aside.
- ❖ Heat your skillet and add the peppers with some of the marinade. Cook for a bit until the onion and peppers are soft.
- ❖ Add the rice to a few serving bowls and top with the bell pepper and onion mixture, salsa and avocado. Add the nutritional yeast and cilantro before serving.

28) Avocado and salmon soup

Preparation time:

Cooking time:

Portions:

Ingredients:

- ✓ Cilantro (2 tablespoons)
- ✓ Crushed pepper (1 teaspoon)
- ✓ Olive oil (1 tablespoon)
- ✓ Flaked salmon (1 can)
- ✓ Salt (.25 tsp.)
- ✓ Cumin (.25 tsp.)
- ✓ Vegetable stock (1.5 c.)

Ingredients:

- ✓ Whole coconut cream (2 tablespoons)
- ✓ Lemon juice (4 tablespoons)
- ✓ Sliced green onion (1 tablespoon)
- ✓ Chopped Shallot (1)
- ✓ Pitted Avocado (3)

Directions:

- ❖ Take out a blender and combine together the salt, cumin, vegetable broth, coconut cream, two tablespoons of lemon juice, green onion, scallion, and avocado.
- ❖ Blend until smooth and then chill in the refrigerator for an hour.

- ❖ Meanwhile, take a bowl and combine together a tablespoon of cilantro, two tablespoons of lemon juice, the pepper, olive oil and salmon.
- ❖ Add the cooled avocado soup to the bowls and top each with the salmon and the rest of the cilantro. Serve immediately.

29) Asian Pumpkin Salad

Preparation time:

Cooking time:

Portions:

Ingredients:
- ✓ Diced avocado (.5)
- ✓ Pomegranate seeds (.25 c.)
- ✓ Lemon juice (1 tablespoon)
- ✓ Sliced cabbage (4 c.)
- ✓ Olive oil (1.5 tablespoons)
- ✓ Diced pumpkin (2 c.)
- ✓ Salt (.5 tsp.)

Directions:
- ❖ Turn on the oven and give it time to heat to 400 degrees. Prepare a baking sheet with baking paper.
- ❖ In a large dish, combine the black and white sesame seeds with the salt, chili flakes, mustard, garlic and cloves.
- ❖ Drizzle the squash with a little olive oil and then roll each cube in the sesame seed mixture, pressing down a little to coat it.

Ingredients:
- ✓ Red pepper flakes (.25 tsp.)
- ✓ Ground mustard (.25 tsp.)
- ✓ Ground Garlic (.25 tsp.)
- ✓ Ground cloves (.25 tsp.)
- ✓ Black sesame seeds (1 tablespoon)
- ✓ White sesame seeds (1 tablespoon)

- ❖ Add the squash to the baking dish and place it in the oven. It will take about half an hour to bake.
- ❖ While the squash is cooking, add the kale to a large bowl and pour in the salt, lemon juice and the rest of the olive oil. Massage the mixture into the kale and then set aside.
- ❖ When the squash is ready, add it on top of the kale and garnish with the avocado and pomegranate seeds before serving.

30) Sweet potato rolls

Preparation time:

Cooking time:

Portions:

Ingredients:
- ✓ Avocado (1)
- ✓ Alfalfa sprouts (1 c.)
- ✓ Sliced red onion (.5)
- ✓ Spinach (1 c.)
- ✓ Cooked quinoa (.5 c.)
- ✓ Swiss chard greens (4)
- ✓ Sweet potato hummus
- ✓ Crushed black pepper (.25 tsp.)

Directions:
- ❖ Take the sweet potatoes and add them to a pan. Cover with water and bring to a boil. When it reaches a boil, reduce the flame and let it cook for a while to make the potatoes tender.
- ❖ When these are ready, drain the water and add them to the food processor along with pepper, salt, cinnamon, chili powder, garlic, lemon juice, olive oil and tahini.

Ingredients:
- ✓ Salt (.25 tsp.)
- ✓ Cinnamon powder (.25 tsp.)
- ✓ Chilli powder (.25 tsp.)
- ✓ Garlic clove (1)
- ✓ Lemon juice (.5)
- ✓ Olive oil (.25 c.)
- ✓ Tahini (.33 c.)
- ✓ Diced sweet potato (1)
- ❖ Process until the mixture is smooth.
- ❖ Lay out each of the green collars and then spread sweet potato hummus on each.
- ❖ Add the avocado, sprouts, onion, spinach and quinoa. Roll everything up and secure with toothpicks. Repeat until the vegetables and filling are done.

31) Spicy cabbage bowl

Preparation time:

Cooking time:

Portions:

Ingredients:
- ✓ Sesame seeds (1 tablespoon)
- ✓ Green onion (.25 c.)
- ✓ Cabbage (2 c.)
- ✓ Coconut amino acids (1 teaspoon)
- ✓ Tamari (2 tablespoons)
- ✓ Chopped kimchi cabbage (1 c.)

Directions:
- ❖ Take out a frying pan and heat the sesame oil in it. When the oil is hot, add together the coconut amino acid, tamari, kimchi, brown rice, garlic and ginger.

Ingredients:
- ✓ Cooked brown rice (1 c.)
- ✓ Chopped garlic (1 teaspoon)
- ✓ Grated ginger (.5 tsp.)
- ✓ Sesame oil (2 tablespoons)

- ❖ After five minutes of cooking these ingredients, add the green onions and cabbage and toss to combine.
- ❖ Cook for a little longer. Then you can garnish the dish with some sesame seeds before serving.

32) Citrus and fennel salad

Preparation time: **Cooking time:**   **Portions:**

Ingredients:

- ✓ Diced avocado (.5)
- ✓ Pomegranate seeds (2 tablespoons)
- ✓ Pepper (.5 tsp.)
- ✓ Salt (.25 tsp.)
- ✓ Olive oil (.25 c.)
- ✓ Orange juice (2 tablespoons)
- ✓ Lemon juice (2 tablespoons)

Directions:

- ❖ To start this recipe, bring out a large bowl and combine together the parsley, mint, fennel slices, grapefruit wedges, and orange wedges. Stir to combine.
- ❖ In another bowl, whisk together the pepper, salt, olive oil, orange juice and lemon juice.

Ingredients:

- ✓ Chopped mint (1 tablespoon)
- ✓ Chopped parsley (.5 c.)
- ✓ Sliced fennel bulbs (2)
- ✓ Red grapefruit segmented (.5)
- ✓ Segmented orange (1)

- ❖ Once combined, pour over the fennel and citrus mixture in the large bowl, stirring to coat.
- ❖ Move to a plate and garnish with the avocado and pomegranate seeds. Serve immediately.

33) Vegan Burger

Preparation time: **Cooking time:**   **Servings: 4 hamburger patties**

Ingredients:

- ✓ 1/4 to 1/2 cup of spring water
- ✓ 1/2 teaspoon of cayenne powder
- ✓ 1/2 teaspoon of ginger powder
- ✓ Grape oil
- ✓ 1 teaspoon of dill
- ✓ 2 teaspoons of sea salt
- ✓ 2 teaspoons of onion powder

Directions:

- ❖ Mix the vegetables and seasonings in a large bowl, then add the flour. Gently add the spring water and stir the mixture until combined. If the mixture is too soft, add more flour.

Ingredients:

- ✓ 2 teaspoons of oregano
- ✓ 2 teaspoons of basil
- ✓ ¼ cup cherry tomatoes, diced
- ✓ 1/2 cup of cabbage, diced
- ✓ 1/2 cup green peppers, diced
- ✓ 1/2 cup onions, diced
- ✓ 1 cup of chickpea flour
- ❖ Divide the dough into 4 meatballs. Cook patties in grapeseed oil, in a skillet over medium heat for about 2 to 3 minutes per side. Continue flipping until the burger is brown on all sides.
- ❖ Serve the burger on a bun and enjoy.

34) Alkaline spicy cabbage

Preparation time: **Cooking time:**   **Servings: 1 portion**

Ingredients:

- ✓ Grape oil
- ✓ 1/4 teaspoon of sea salt
- ✓ 1 teaspoon crushed red pepper

Directions:

- ❖ First wash the cabbage well and then fold each cabbage leaf in half. Cut off and discard the stems. Cut the prepared cabbage into bite-size portions and use the salad spinner to remove the water.
- ❖ In a wok, add 2 tablespoons of grapeseed oil and heat the oil over high heat.

Ingredients:

- ✓ 1/4 cup red bell bell pepper, diced
- ✓ 1/4 cup onion, diced
- ✓ 1 bunch of cabbage

- ❖ Fry the peppers and onions in the oil for about 2-3 minutes and then season with a little sea salt.
- ❖ Lower the heat and add the cabbage, cover the wok with a lid and simmer for about 5 minutes.
- ❖ Open the lid and add the crushed pepper, mix well and cover again. Cook until tender, or about 3 more minutes.

35) Electric Salad

Preparation time: **Cooking time:** **Servings: 4**

Ingredients:
- ✓ 3 jalapenos
- ✓ 2 red onions
- ✓ 1 orange bell pepper
- ✓ 1 yellow bell pepper
- ✓ 1 cup cherry tomatoes, chopped

Directions:
- ❖ First wash and rinse the ingredients well. Dry the ingredients and then cut them into bite-size pieces, or as required.

Ingredients:
- ✓ 1 bunch of cabbage
- ✓ 1 handful of romaine lettuce
- ✓ Extra virgin olive oil
- ✓ Juice of 1 lime

- ❖ Place ingredients in a bowl and drizzle with olive oil and lime juice to your preferred taste.

36) Kale salad

Preparation time: **Cooking time:** **Servings: 2**

Ingredients:
- ✓ 1/4 teaspoon of cayenne
- ✓ 1/2 teaspoon of sea salt
- ✓ 1/2 cup of cooked chickpeas
- ✓ 1/2 cup of red onions
- ✓ 1/2 cup sliced red, orange, yellow and green peppers
- ✓ 4 cups chopped cabbage

Directions:
- ❖ In a bowl, mix all the ingredients for the coleslaw and toss.

Ingredients:
- ✓ 1/2 cup alkaline garlic sauce (recipe included).
- ✓ Alkaline Garlic Sauce
- ✓ 1/4 teaspoon of dill
- ✓ 1/4 teaspoon of sea salt
- ✓ 1/2 teaspoon of ginger
- ✓ 1 tablespoon of onion powder
- ✓ 1/4 cup shallots, chopped
- ✓ 1 cup of grape oil
- ❖ Prepare the dressing by mixing the ingredients for the "Alkaline Electric Garlic Sauce".
- ❖ Drizzle with half a cup of sauce and then serve.

37) Walnut, date, orange and cabbage salad

Preparation time: **Cooking time:** **Servings: 2**

Ingredients:
- ✓ /2 red onion, very thinly sliced
- ✓ 2 bunches of cabbage, or 6 full cups of sprouts
- ✓ 6 medjool dates, pitted
- ✓ 1/3 cup whole walnuts
- ✓ For the dressing

Directions:
- ❖ Preheat the oven to 375 degrees F and then place the walnuts on a baking sheet. Roast the walnuts for about 7-8 minutes, or until the skin begins to darken and crack.
- ❖ Once done, transfer the walnuts while still warm and let them steam for 15 minutes wrapped in a kitchen towel.
- ❖ Once cooled, squeeze and turn firmly to remove the skin, all still wrapped in the towel.
- ❖ In a food processor, place the pitted dates along with the walnuts and puree until fully blended and finely chopped. Set aside to cover the salad.

Ingredients:
- ✓ 5 tablespoons of olive oil
- ✓ Pinch of coarse salt
- ✓ 1 medjool date
- ✓ 4 tablespoons of freshly squeezed orange juice
- ✓ 2 tablespoons of lime juice
- ❖ Then wash, dry and cut the cabbage and place in a large bowl. Thinly slice the onion and add it to the bowl.
- ❖ Now prepare the dressing by combining the ingredients for the "dressing" in the blender apart from the olive oil.
- ❖ Blend the mixture to break up the dates and then pour in the oil in a steady stream to emulsify the dressing.
- ❖ Finally, toss the cabbage and onion mixture with the orange and walnut dressing.
- ❖ Move to a serving bowl and sprinkle with the walnut and date mixture. Enjoy!

38) Tomatoes with basil-snack

Preparation time: **Cooking time:**   **Servings: 1 portion**

Ingredients:

- ¼ teaspoon of sea salt
- 2 tablespoons of lemon juice
- 2 tablespoons of olive oil

Directions:

- ❖ Start by slicing the cherry tomatoes and placing them in a medium sized bowl.
- ❖ Then finely chop your basil and add it to the bowl of tomatoes.

Ingredients:

- ¼ cup basil, fresh
- 1 cup chopped tomatoes, cherry or Roma

- ❖ Drizzle the tomatoes and basil with a little olive oil and lemon juice.
- ❖ Add a little sea salt to taste.
- ❖ Serve.

39) Pasta with spelt, zucchini and eggplant

Preparation time: **Cooking time:**   **Servings: 4**

Ingredients:

- 2 teaspoons of dried basil leaves
- 1 teaspoon of oregano
- 2/3 cup vegetable broth
- 2/3 cup of dried and diced cherry tomatoes
- 1 large zucchini, diced
- 3 medium-sized, ripe cherry tomatoes, diced

Directions:

- ❖ Over medium heat, heat a little oil in a skillet and then sauté the eggplant, ginger and onion for about 8-10 minutes, stirring constantly.
- ❖ Then add the oregano, tomatoes and zucchini and let cook for 6-8 minutes, stirring occasionally.

Ingredients:

- 2-3 ginger, crushed
- 1-2 white onions, finely chopped
- 3 tablespoons of cold-pressed extra virgin olive oil
- 1 large eggplant cut into cubes
- 300g of spelt pasta
- Sea salt to taste
- ❖ Now heat the water and cook the pasta until it is firm to the bite, and then add the vegetable broth to the pan.
- ❖ Season with fresh pepper, salt and dried basil. Allow the mixture to simmer for a few minutes, covered.
- ❖ Once cooked, you can serve the sauce over pasta and garnish with fresh basil leaves.

40) Alkalizing millet dish

Preparation time: **Cooking time:**   **Servings: 2**

Ingredients:

- 1/2 teaspoon of sea salt
- 2 1/2 cups of water

Directions:

- ❖ In a pot with an airtight lid, add the millet and then sauté over medium heat, stirring constantly.
- ❖ As soon as the millet turns golden brown, add the sea salt and water and cover the ingredients with a lid.
- ❖ Then bring the mixture to a boil and let it simmer until all the water has been absorbed, or for about 25-35 minutes.

Ingredients:

- 1 cup millet

- ❖ Alternatively, you can cook on an electric stove. Just cover the lid and bring to a boil, simmer for a couple of minutes and then turn off the stove.
- ❖ Allow the contents to cool for about 30 minutes with the lid on to allow the millet to dry out.
- ❖ Then serve and enjoy the millet.

Alkaline Diet Dinner Recipes

41) Mixed stew of spicy vegetables

Preparation time: 20 minutes   **Cooking time**: 35 minutes   **Servings: 8**

Ingredients:

- ✓ 2 tablespoons of coconut oil
- ✓ 1 large sweet onion, chopped
- ✓ 1 medium parsnip, peeled and chopped
- ✓ 3 tablespoons of homemade tomato paste
- ✓ 2 large garlic cloves, minced
- ✓ ½ teaspoon of cinnamon powder
- ✓ ½ teaspoon ground ginger
- ✓ 1 teaspoon of ground cumin
- ✓ ¼ teaspoon cayenne pepper

Directions:

- ❖ In a large soup pot, melt the coconut oil over medium-high heat and sauté the onion for about 5 minutes.
- ❖ Add the parsnips and sauté for about 3 minutes.
- ❖ Add the tomato paste, garlic and spices and sauté for 2 minutes.

Ingredients:

- ✓ 2 medium carrots, peeled and chopped
- ✓ 2 medium purple potatoes, peeled and cut into pieces
- ✓ 2 medium sweet potatoes, peeled and cut into pieces
- ✓ 4 cups of homemade vegetable broth
- ✓ 2 tablespoons fresh lemon juice
- ✓ 2 cups fresh cabbage, hard ribs removed and chopped
- ✓ ¼ cup fresh parsley leaves, chopped

- ❖ Stir in the carrots, potatoes, sweet potatoes and broth and bring to a boil.
- ❖ Reduce heat to medium-low and simmer, covered for about 20 minutes.
- ❖ Add the lemon juice and cabbage and simmer for 5 minutes.
- ❖ Serve with a garnish of parsley.

42) Mixed vegetable stew with herbs

Preparation time: 15 minutes   **Cooking time**: 2¼ hours   **Servings: 8**

Ingredients:

- ✓ 2 tablespoons of coconut oil
- ✓ 1 medium yellow onion, chopped
- ✓ 2 cups celery, chopped
- ✓ ½ teaspoon of minced garlic
- ✓ 3 cups fresh cabbage, hard ribs removed and chopped
- ✓ ½ cup fresh mushrooms, sliced
- ✓ 2½ cups tomatoes, finely chopped
- ✓ 1 teaspoon dried rosemary, crushed

Directions:

- ❖ In a large skillet, melt the coconut oil over medium heat and sauté the onion, celery and garlic for about 5 minutes.
- ❖ Add the rest of all ingredients and stir to combine.
- ❖ Increase heat to high and bring to a boil.
- ❖ Cook for about 10 minutes.

Ingredients:

- ✓ 1 teaspoon dried sage, crushed
- ✓ 1 teaspoon dried oregano, crushed
- ✓ Sea salt and freshly ground black pepper, to taste
- ✓ 2 cups of homemade vegetable broth
- ✓ 3-4 cups of alkaline water
- ✓ ¼ cup fresh parsley, chopped

- ❖ Reduce heat to medium and cook, covered for about 15 minutes.
- ❖ Uncover the pan and cook for about 15 minutes, stirring occasionally.
- ❖ Now, reduce the heat to low and simmer, covered for about 1 1/2 hours.
- ❖ Serve warm with a garnish of parsley.

43) Tofu and bell pepper stew

Preparation time: 15 minutes   **Cooking time**: 15 minutes   **Servings: 6**

Ingredients:

- ✓ 2 tablespoons of garlic
- ✓ 1 jalapeño bell pepper, seeded and chopped
- ✓ 1 (16-ounce) can of roasted, rinsed, drained and chopped red peppers
- ✓ 2 cups of homemade vegetable broth
- ✓ 2 cups of alkaline water

Directions:

- ❖ In a food processor, add the garlic, jalapeño bell pepper and roasted red peppers and pulse until smooth.
- ❖ In a large skillet, add the pepper puree, broth and water over medium-high heat and bring to a boil.
- ❖ Add the peppers and tofu and stir to combine.

Ingredients:

- ✓ 1 medium green bell pepper, seeded and thinly sliced
- ✓ 1 medium red bell pepper, seeded and thinly sliced
- ✓ 1 (16-ounce) package of extra-firm tofu, drained and diced
- ✓ 10 ounces of frozen sprouts, thawed
- ✓ Sea salt and freshly ground black pepper, to taste

- ❖ Reduce the heat to medium and cook for about 5 minutes.
- ❖ Stir in the cabbage and cook for about 5 minutes.
- ❖ Add the salt and black pepper and remove from heat.
- ❖ Serve hot.

44) Roasted Pumpkin Curry

Preparation time: 15 minutes **Cooking time**: 35 minutes **Servings: 4**

Ingredients:

For the roasted squash:
- ✓ 1 medium-sized sugar pumpkin, peeled and cut into cubes
- ✓ Sea salt, to taste
- ✓ 1 teaspoon of olive oil

For Curry:
- ✓ 1 teaspoon of olive oil
- ✓ 1 onion, chopped
- ✓ 1 tablespoon fresh ginger root, peeled and chopped

Directions:

- ❖ Preheat oven to 400 degrees F. Line a large baking sheet with baking paper.
- ❖ In a large bowl, add all the ingredients for the roasted squash and stir to coat well.
- ❖ Arrange the pumpkins on the prepared baking sheet in a single layer.
- ❖ Roast for about 20-25 minutes, turning once halfway through.

Ingredients:

- ✓ 1 tablespoon chopped garlic
- ✓ 1 cup unsweetened coconut milk
- ✓ 2 cups of vegetable broth
- ✓ 1 teaspoon of ground cumin
- ✓ ½ teaspoon ground turmeric
- ✓ Sea salt and freshly ground black pepper, to taste
- ✓ 1 tablespoon fresh lime juice
- ✓ 2 tablespoons fresh parsley, chopped

- ❖ Meanwhile, for the curry: in a large skillet, heat the oil over medium-high heat and sauté the onion for about 4-5 minutes.
- ❖ Add the ginger and garlic and sauté for about 1 minute.
- ❖ Add the coconut milk, broth, spices, salt and black pepper and bring to a boil.
- ❖ Reduce the heat to low and simmer for about 10 minutes.
- ❖ Add the roasted squash and simmer for another 10 minutes.
- ❖ Serve warm with a garnish of parsley.

45) Lentils, vegetables and apple curry

Preparation time: 20 minutes **Cooking time:** 1 hour and a half **Servings: 6**

Ingredients:

- ✓ 8 cups of alkaline water
- ✓ ½ teaspoon ground turmeric
- ✓ 1 cup brown lentils
- ✓ 1 cup of red lentils
- ✓ 1 tablespoon of olive oil
- ✓ 1 large white onion, chopped
- ✓ 3 garlic cloves, minced
- ✓ 2 tomatoes, seeded and chopped

Directions:

- ❖ In a large skillet, add the water, turmeric and lentils over high heat and bring to a boil.
- ❖ Reduce heat to medium-low and simmer, covered for about 30 minutes.
- ❖ Drain the lentils, reserving 2½ cups of the cooking liquid.
- ❖ Meanwhile, in another large skillet, heat the oil over medium heat and sauté the onion for about 2-3 minutes.
- ❖ Add the garlic and sauté for about 1 minute.
- ❖ Add the tomatoes and cook for about 5 minutes.

Ingredients:

- ✓ ¼ teaspoon ground cloves
- ✓ 2 teaspoons of ground cumin
- ✓ 2 carrots, peeled and cut into pieces
- ✓ 2 potatoes, peeled and cut into pieces
- ✓ 2 cups pumpkin, peeled, seeded and cut into 1-inch cubes
- ✓ 1 granny smith apple, cored and chopped
- ✓ 2 cups fresh cabbage, hard ribs removed and chopped
- ✓ Sea salt and freshly ground black pepper, to taste
- ❖ Stir in the spices and cook for about 1 minute.
- ❖ Add the carrots, potatoes, squash, cooked lentils and reserved cooking liquid and bring to a gentle boil.
- ❖ Reduce heat to medium-low and simmer, covered for about 40-45 minutes or until desired doneness of vegetables.
- ❖ Add the apple and cabbage and simmer for about 15 minutes.
- ❖ Add the salt and black pepper and remove from heat.
- ❖ Serve hot.

46) Curried red beans

Preparation time: 15 minutes **Cooking time:** 25 minutes **Servings: 6**

Ingredients:

- ✓ 4 tablespoons of olive oil
- ✓ 1 medium onion, finely chopped
- ✓ 2 garlic cloves, minced
- ✓ 2 tablespoons of fresh ginger root, peeled and chopped
- ✓ 1 teaspoon of ground coriander
- ✓ 1 teaspoon of ground cumin
- ✓ ½ teaspoon ground turmeric

Directions:

- ❖ In a large skillet, heat the oil over medium heat and sauté the onion, garlic and ginger for about 6-8 minutes.
- ❖ Stir in the spices and cook for about 1-2 minutes.

Ingredients:

- ✓ ¼ teaspoon cayenne pepper
- ✓ Sea salt and freshly ground black pepper, to taste
- ✓ 2 large plum tomatoes, finely chopped
- ✓ 3 cups of cooked red beans
- ✓ 2 cups of alkaline water
- ✓ ¼ cup fresh parsley, chopped

- ❖ Add the tomatoes, beans and water and bring to a boil over high heat.
- ❖ Reduce heat to medium and simmer for 10-15 minutes or until desired thickness.
- ❖ Serve warm with a garnish of parsley.

47) Lentil and Carrot Chili

Preparation time: 15 minutes

Cooking time: 2 hours and 40 minutes

Servings: 8

Ingredients:
- ✓ 2 teaspoons of olive oil
- ✓ 1 large onion, chopped
- ✓ 3 medium carrots, peeled and chopped
- ✓ 4 celery stalks, chopped
- ✓ 2 garlic cloves, minced
- ✓ • 1 jalapeño bell pepper, seeded and chopped
- ✓ ½ tablespoon dried thyme, crushed
- ✓ 1 tablespoon of chipotle chili powder

Ingredients:
- ✓ ½ tablespoon of cayenne pepper
- ✓ 1½ tablespoons ground coriander
- ✓ 1½ tablespoons of ground cumin
- ✓ 1 teaspoon ground turmeric
- ✓ Sea salt and freshly ground black pepper, to taste
- ✓ 1 pound red lentils, rinsed
- ✓ 8 cups of homemade vegetable broth
- ✓ ½ cup shallots, chopped

Directions:
- ❖ In a large skillet, heat the oil over medium heat and sauté the onion, carrot and celery for about 5 minutes.
- ❖ Add the garlic, jalapeño pepper, thyme and spices and sauté for about 1 minute.

- ❖ Add the lentils and broth and bring to a boil.
- ❖ Reduce heat to low and simmer, covered for about 2-2½ hours.
- ❖ Remove from heat and serve hot with a scallion garnish.

48) Black beans with chilli

Preparation time: 15 minutes

Cooking time: 2 hours and 5 minutes

Servings: 5

Ingredients:
- ✓ 2 tablespoons of olive oil
- ✓ 1 onion, chopped
- ✓ 1 large green bell pepper, seeded and sliced
- ✓ 4 garlic cloves, minced
- ✓ 2 jalapeño peppers, sliced
- ✓ 1 teaspoon of ground cumin
- ✓ 1 teaspoon of cayenne pepper

Ingredients:
- ✓ 1 tablespoon of red chili powder
- ✓ 1 teaspoon of paprika
- ✓ 2 cups of tomatoes, finely chopped
- ✓ 4 cups of cooked black beans
- ✓ 2 cups of homemade vegetable broth
- ✓ Sea salt and freshly ground black pepper, to taste
- ✓ ¼ cup fresh parsley, chopped
- ❖ Reduce heat to medium-low and simmer, covered for about 1½-2 hours.
- ❖ Season with the salt and black pepper and remove from heat.
- ❖ Serve warm with a garnish of parsley.

Directions:
- ❖ In a large skillet, heat the oil over medium-high heat and sauté the onion and peppers for 3-4 minutes.
- ❖ Add the garlic, jalapeño peppers and spices and sauté for about 1 minute.
- ❖ Add the remaining ingredients and bring to a boil.

49) Cook mixed vegetables

Preparation time: 15 minutes

Cooking time: 20 minutes

Servings: 4

Ingredients:
- ✓ 1 small zucchini, chopped
- ✓ 1 small summer squash, chopped
- ✓ 1 diced eggplant
- ✓ 1 red bell pepper, seeded and diced
- ✓ 1 green bell pepper, seeded and diced

Ingredients:
- ✓ 1 onion, thinly sliced
- ✓ 1 tablespoon of pure maple syrup
- ✓ 2 tablespoons of olive oil
- ✓ Sea salt and freshly ground black pepper, to taste

- ❖ Transfer the vegetable mixture to the prepared baking dish.
- ❖ Bake for about 15-20 minutes.
- ❖ Remove from oven and serve immediately.

Directions:
- ❖ Preheat oven to 375 degrees F. Lightly grease a large baking dish.
- ❖ In a large bowl, add all ingredients and mix well.

50) Vegetarian Ratatouille

Preparation time: 20 minutes   **Cooking time**: 45 minutes   **Servings: 4**

Ingredients:

- ✓ 6 ounces of homemade tomato paste
- ✓ 3 tablespoons of olive oil, divided by
- ✓ ½ onion, chopped
- ✓ 3 tablespoons minced garlic
- ✓ Sea salt and freshly ground black pepper, to taste
- ✓ 1 zucchini, cut into thin circles

Directions:

- ❖ Preheat the oven to 375 degrees F.
- ❖ In a bowl, add tomato paste, 1 tablespoon oil, onion, garlic, salt and black pepper and mix well.
- ❖ In the bottom of a 10x10-inch baking dish, spread tomato paste mixture evenly.
- ❖ Arrange the vegetable slices alternately, starting at the outer edge of the pan and working concentrically toward the center.

Ingredients:

- ✓ 1 yellow pumpkin, cut in thin circles
- ✓ 1 eggplant, cut into thin circles
- ✓ 1 red bell pepper, with seeds and cut into thin rounds
- ✓ 1 yellow bell pepper, with seeds and cut into thin rounds
- ✓ 1 tablespoon fresh thyme leaves, chopped
- ✓ 1 tablespoon fresh lemon juice
- ❖ Drizzle the vegetables with the remaining oil and sprinkle with salt and black pepper, followed by the thyme.
- ❖ Arrange a piece of parchment paper over the vegetables.
- ❖ Bake for about 45 minutes.
- ❖ Remove from oven and serve hot.

51) Quinoa with vegetables

Preparation time: 15 minutes   **Cooking time**: 26 minutes   **Servings: 4**

Ingredients:

- For roasted mushrooms:
- ✓ 2 cups of small fresh Baby Bella mushrooms
- ✓ 1 tablespoon of olive oil
- ✓ Sea salt, to taste

- For the quinoa:
- ✓ 2 cups of alkaline water
- ✓ 1 cup red quinoa, rinsed
- ✓ 2 tablespoons fresh parsley, chopped

Directions:

- ❖ Preheat oven to 425 degrees F. Line a large rimmed baking sheet with parchment paper.
- ❖ In a bowl, add the mushrooms, oil and salt and stir to coat well.
- ❖ Arrange the mushrooms on the prepared baking sheet in a single layer.
- ❖ Roast for about 15-18 minutes, tossing once halfway through cooking.
- ❖ Meanwhile, for the quinoa: in a skillet, add the water and quinoa over medium-high heat and bring to a boil.
- ❖ Reduce the heat to low and simmer, covered for about 15-20 minutes or until all the liquid is absorbed.
- ❖ Remove from heat and set pan aside, covered for about 5 minutes.
- ❖ Uncover the pan and with a fork, stir in the quinoa.

Ingredients:

- ✓ 1 garlic clove chopped
- ✓ 1 tablespoon of olive oil
- ✓ 2 teaspoons of fresh lemon juice
- ✓ Sea salt and freshly ground black pepper, to taste

- For the broccoli:
- ✓ 1 cup of broccoli florets
- ✓ 2 tablespoons of olive oil

- ❖ Stir in the parsley, garlic, oil, lemon juice, salt and black pepper and set aside to cool completely.
- ❖ Meanwhile, for the broccoli: in a pot of water, arrange a steamer basket and bring to a boil.
- ❖ Place the broccoli florets in the basket of the steamer and steam, covered for about 5-6 minutes.
- ❖ Drain broccoli florets well.
- ❖ Transfer the broccoli florets to the bowl with the quinoa and mushrooms and stir to combine.
- ❖ Drizzle with the oil and serve immediately.

52) Lentils with cabbage

Preparation time: 15 minutes   **Cooking time**: 20 minutes   **Servings: 6**

Ingredients:
- ✓ 1½ cups of red lentils
- ✓ 1½ cups homemade vegetable broth
- ✓ 1½ tablespoons of olive oil
- ✓ ½ cup onion, chopped
- ✓ 1 teaspoon fresh ginger, chopped

Directions:
- ❖ In a skillet, add the broth and lentils over medium-high heat and bring to a boil.
- ❖ Reduce heat and simmer, covered for about 20 minutes or until almost all liquid is absorbed.
- ❖ Remove from heat and set aside covered.

Ingredients:
- ✓ 2 garlic cloves, minced
- ✓ 1½ cups tomato, chopped
- ✓ 6 cups fresh cabbage, hard ribs removed and chopped
- ✓ Sea salt and ground black pepper, to taste

- ❖ Meanwhile, in a large skillet, heat the oil over medium heat and sauté the onion for about 5-6 minutes.
- ❖ Add the ginger and garlic and sauté for about 1 minute.
- ❖ Add the tomatoes and cabbage and cook for about 4-5 minutes.
- ❖ Add the lentils, salt and black pepper and remove from heat.
- ❖ Remove from heat and serve hot.

53) Lentils with tomatoes

Preparation time: 15 minutes   **Cooking time**: 55 minutes   **Servings: 4**

Ingredients:
- ✓ For the tomato puree:
- ✓ 1 cup tomatoes, chopped
- ✓ 1 garlic clove, minced
- ✓ 1 green chilli chopped
- ✓ ¼ cup alkaline water

- For the lentils:
- ✓ 1 cup of red lentils
- ✓ 3 cups of alkaline water

Directions:
- ❖ To tomato paste in a blender, add all ingredients and pulse until it forms a smooth puree. Set aside.
- ❖ In a large skillet, add 3 cups of water and the lentils over high heat and bring to a boil.
- ❖ Reduce heat to medium-low and simmer, covered for about 15-20 minutes or until quite tender.
- ❖ Drain lentils well.

Ingredients:
- ✓ 1 tablespoon of olive oil
- ✓ ½ medium white onion, chopped
- ✓ ½ teaspoon of ground cumin
- ✓ ½ teaspoon of cayenne pepper
- ✓ ¼ teaspoon ground turmeric
- ✓ ¼ cup tomato, chopped
- ✓ ¼ cup fresh parsley leaves, chopped

- ❖ In a large skillet, heat the oil over medium heat and sauté the onion for about 6-7 minutes.
- ❖ Add the spices and sauté for about 1 minute.
- ❖ Add the tomato puree and cook, stirring for about 5-7 minutes.
- ❖ Stir in lentils and cook for about 4-5 minutes or until desired degree of doneness.
- ❖ Stir in chopped tomato and immediately remove from heat.
- ❖ Serve warm with a garnish of parsley.

54) Spicy baked beans

Preparation time: 15 minutes   **Cooking time**: 2 hours and 5 minutes   **Servings: 4**

Ingredients:

- ½ pound of dried red beans, soaked overnight and drained
- 1¼ tablespoons of olive oil
- 1 small yellow onion, chopped
- 4 garlic cloves, minced
- 1 teaspoon dried thyme, crushed
- ½ teaspoon of ground cumin
- ½ teaspoon of red pepper flakes, crushed

Directions:

- In a large pot of boiling water, add the beans and bring to a boil.
- Reduce heat to low and cook, covered for about 1 hour.
- Remove from heat and drain beans well.
- Preheat the oven to 325 degrees F.
- In a large ovenproof skillet, heat the oil over medium heat and sauté the onion for about 4 minutes.

Ingredients:

- ¼ teaspoon of smoked paprika
- 1 tablespoon fresh lemon juice
- 1 cup of homemade tomato sauce
- 1 cup of homemade vegetable broth
- Sea salt and freshly ground black pepper, to taste

- Add the garlic, thyme and spices and sauté for about 1 minute.
- Add the cooked beans and other ingredients and immediately remove from heat.
- Cover the pan and bake for about 1 hour.
- Remove from oven and serve hot.

55) Chickpeas with pumpkin

Preparation time: 20 minutes   **Cooking time**: 35 minutes   **Servings: 4**

Ingredients:

- 1 tablespoon of olive oil
- 1 onion, chopped
- 2 garlic cloves, minced
- 1 green chili pepper, seedless and finely chopped
- 1 teaspoon of ground cumin
- ½ teaspoon of ground coriander
- 1 teaspoon of red chili powder

Directions:

- In a large skillet, heat the oil over medium-high heat and sauté the onion for about 5-7 minutes.
- Add the garlic, green chiles and spices and sauté for about 1 minute.
- Add tomatoes and cook for 2-3 minutes, mashing with the back of a spoon.

Ingredients:

- 2 cups fresh tomatoes, finely chopped
- 2 pounds of pumpkin, peeled and diced
- 2 cups of homemade vegetable broth
- 2 cups of cooked chickpeas
- 2 tablespoons fresh lemon juice
- Sea salt and freshly ground black pepper, to taste
- 2 tablespoons fresh parsley leaves, chopped
- Add the squash and cook for about 3-4 minutes, stirring occasionally.
- Add the broth and bring to a boil.
- Reduce the heat to low and simmer for about 10 minutes.
- Stir in the chickpeas and simmer for about 10 minutes.
- Add the lemon juice, salt and black pepper and remove from heat.
- Serve warm with a garnish of parsley.

56) Chickpeas with cabbage

Preparation time: 15 minutes   **Cooking time**: 18 minutes   **Servings: 6**

Ingredients:

- 2 tablespoons of olive oil
- 1 medium onion, chopped
- 4 garlic cloves, minced
- 1 teaspoon dried thyme, crushed
- 1 teaspoon dried oregano, crushed
- ½ teaspoon of paprika
- 1 cup of tomato, finely chopped

Directions:

- In a large skillet, heat the oil over medium heat and sauté the onion for about 8-9 minutes.
- Add the garlic, herbs and paprika and sauté for about 1 minute.
- Add the cabbage and water and cook for about 2-3 minutes.

Ingredients:

- 2 ½ cups cooked chickpeas
- 4 cups fresh cabbage, hard ribs removed and chopped
- 2 tablespoons of alkaline water
- 2 tablespoons fresh lemon juice
- Sea salt and freshly ground black pepper, to taste
- 3 tablespoons fresh basil, chopped
- Add the tomatoes and chickpeas and cook for about 3-5 minutes.
- Add the lemon juice, salt and black pepper and remove from heat.
- Serve warm with the basil garnish.

57) Stuffed cabbage rolls

Preparation time: 15 minutes   **Cooking time:** 15 minutes   **Servings: 4**

Ingredients:

For filling:
- ✓ 1½ cups fresh button mushrooms, chopped
- ✓ 3¼ cups zucchini, chopped
- ✓ 1 cup red bell pepper, seeded and chopped
- ✓ 1 cup green bell pepper, seeded and chopped
- ✓ ½ teaspoon dried thyme, crushed
- ✓ ½ teaspoon dried marjoram, crushed
- ✓ ½ teaspoon dried basil, crushed

Directions:
- ❖ Preheat oven to 400 degrees F. Lightly grease a 13x9-inch casserole dish.
- ❖ For the filling: in a large skillet, add all ingredients except lemon juice over medium heat and bring to a boil.
- ❖ Reduce heat to low and simmer, covered for about 5 minutes.
- ❖ Remove from heat and set aside for about 5 minutes.
- ❖ Add the lemon juice and stir to combine.
- ❖ Meanwhile, for the rolls: in a large pot of boiling water, add the cabbage leaves and boil for about 2-4 minutes.
- ❖ Drain the cabbage leaves well.
- ❖ Thoroughly dry each cabbage leaf with paper towels.
- ❖ Arrange the cabbage leaves on a smooth surface.
- ❖ Using a knife, make a V-shaped cut in each leaf by cutting through the thick vein.

Ingredients:
- ✓ Sea salt and freshly ground black pepper, to taste
- ✓ ½ cup homemade vegetable broth
- ✓ 2 teaspoons of fresh lemon juice

For rolls:
- ✓ 8 large cabbage leaves, rinsed
- ✓ 8 ounces of homemade tomato sauce
- ✓ 3 tablespoons fresh parsley, chopped

- ❖ Carefully overlap the cut ends of each leaf.
- ❖ Place the filling mixture evenly on each leaf and fold in the sides.
- ❖ Then, roll up each leaf to seal in the filling and then, secure each leaf with toothpicks.
- ❖ In the bottom of the prepared casserole dish, place 1/3 cup of the tomato sauce evenly.
- ❖ Arrange cabbage rolls on top of sauce in a single layer and top with remaining sauce evenly.
- ❖ Cover the casserole dish and cook for about 15 minutes.
- ❖ Remove from oven and set aside, uncovered for about 5 minutes.
- ❖ Serve warm with a garnish of parsley.

58) Green beans and mushrooms in casserole

Preparation time: 20 minutes   **Cooking time:** 20 minutes   **Servings: 6**

Ingredients:

For the onion slices:
- ✓ ½ cup yellow onion, very thinly sliced
- ✓ ¼ cup almond flour
- ✓ 1/8 teaspoon of garlic powder
- ✓ Sea salt and freshly ground black pepper, to taste

For the casserole:
- ✓ 1 pound fresh green beans, chopped
- ✓ 1 tablespoon of olive oil

Directions:
- ❖ Preheat the oven to 350 degrees F.
- ❖ For the onion slices: in a bowl, place all ingredients and mix to coat well.
- ❖ Arrange the onion slices on a large baking sheet in a single layer and set aside.
- ❖ For the casserole: in a pot of boiling salted water, add the green beans and cook for about 5 minutes.
- ❖ Drain green beans and transfer to a bowl of ice water.
- ❖ Again, drain well and transfer to a large bowl. Set aside.
- ❖ In a large skillet, heat the oil over medium-high heat and sauté the mushrooms, onion, garlic powder, salt and black pepper for about 2-3 minutes.

Ingredients:
- ✓ 8 ounces fresh cremini mushrooms, sliced
- ✓ ½ cup yellow onion, thinly sliced
- ✓ 1/8 teaspoon of garlic powder
- ✓ Sea salt and freshly ground black pepper, to taste
- ✓ 1 teaspoon fresh thyme, chopped
- ✓ ½ cup homemade vegetable broth
- ✓ ½ cup of coconut cream

- ❖ Stir in the thyme and broth and cook for about 3-5 minutes or until all the liquid is absorbed.
- ❖ Remove from heat and transfer the mushroom mixture to the bowl with the green beans.
- ❖ Add the coconut cream and stir to combine well.
- ❖ Transfer the mixture to a 10-inch casserole dish.
- ❖ Place the casserole dish and onion slice pan in the oven.
- ❖ Bake for about 15-17 minutes.
- ❖ Remove the pan and sheet from the oven and let cool for about 5 minutes before serving.
- ❖ Top the casserole with the crispy onion slices evenly.
- ❖ Cut into 6 equal-sized portions and serve.

59) Meatloaf of wild rice and lentils

Preparation time: 20 minutes   **Cooking time:** 1 hour and 50 minutes   **Servings: 8**

Ingredients:

- ✓ 1¾ cups plus 2 tablespoons of alkaline water, divided
- ✓ ½ cup wild rice
- ✓ ½ cup of brown lentils
- ✓ Pinch of sea salt
- ✓ ½ teaspoon of sodium-free Italian seasoning
- ✓ 1 medium yellow onion, chopped
- ✓ 1 celery stalk, chopped
- ✓ 6 cremini mushrooms, chopped

Directions:

- ❖ In a saucepan, add 1¾ cups water, the rice, lentils, salt and Italian seasoning and bring to a boil over medium-high heat.
- ❖ Reduce the heat to low and simmer covered for about 45 minutes.
- ❖ Remove from heat and set aside, covered for at least 10 minutes.
- ❖ Preheat oven to 350 degrees F. Line a 9x5-inch baking dish with baking paper.
- ❖ In a skillet, heat the remaining water over medium heat and sauté the onion, celery, mushrooms and garlic for about 4-5 minutes.
- ❖ Remove from heat and allow to cool slightly.
- ❖ In a large bowl, add the oats, pecans, tomato sauce and fresh herbs and stir until well combined.

Ingredients:

- ✓ 4 garlic cloves, minced
- ✓ ¾ cup rolled oats
- ✓ ½ cup pecans, finely chopped
- ✓ ¾ cup of homemade tomato sauce
- ✓ ½ teaspoon of red pepper flakes, crushed
- ✓ 1 teaspoon fresh rosemary, chopped
- ✓ 2 teaspoons fresh thyme, chopped

- ❖ Combine the rice mixture and vegetable mixture with the oat mixture and mix well.
- ❖ In a blender, add the mixture and pulse until it forms a chunky mixture.
- ❖ Transfer the mixture to the prepared baking dish evenly.
- ❖ With a piece of foil, cover the pan and bake for about 40 minutes.
- ❖ Uncover and bake for about 15-20 minutes more or until the top turns golden brown.
- ❖ Remove from oven and set aside for about 5-10 minutes before slicing.
- ❖ Cut into slices of desired size and serve

60) Vegetable soup and spelt noodles

Preparation time: 5 minutes   **Cooking time:** 12 minutes   **Servings: 2**

Ingredients:

- ✓ ½ onion, peeled, cut into cubes
- ✓ ½ green bell pepper, chopped
- ✓ ½ zucchini, grated
- ✓ 4 ounces (113 g) sliced mushrooms, chopped
- ✓ ½ cup of cherry tomatoes
- ✓ ¼ cup of basil leaves

Directions:

- ❖ Take a medium saucepan, put it over medium heat, add the oil and when hot, add the onion and then cook for 3 minutes or more until tender.
- ❖ Add the cherry tomatoes, bell bell pepper and mushrooms, stir until combined and continue cooking for 3 minutes until soft.
- ❖ Add the grated zucchini, season with salt, cayenne pepper, pour in the water and bring the mixture to a boil.

Ingredients:

- ✓ 1 package of spelt tagliatelle, cooked
- ✓ ¼ teaspoon salt
- ✓ ⅛ teaspoon of cayenne pepper
- ✓ ½ key lime, squeezed
- ✓ 1 tablespoon of grape oil
- ✓ 2 cups of spring water
- ❖ Then, turn the heat down to low, add the cooked noodles and simmer the soup for 5 minutes.
- ❖ When finished, pour soup into two bowls, top with basil leaves, drizzle with lime juice and serve.

61) Quinoa Salad

Preparation time: **Cooking time:** **Servings: 2**

Ingredients:

- ✓ 1 cup quinoa, cooked
- ✓ 1 garlic clove, minced
- ✓ 1 cucumber, chopped
- ✓ 1 cup of fresh arugula leaves
- ✓ 1 red bell pepper, chopped
- ✓ 1 large avocado, peeled, pitted and diced

Directions:

- ❖ Just combine all the ingredients in a large salad bowl.

Ingredients:

- ✓ 2 tablespoons of chia seeds (optional)
- ✓ 2 tablespoons of olive oil
- ✓ 2 tablespoons of coconut milk (I think)
- ✓ Himalayan salt and black pepper to taste
- ✓ Juice of 1 lime or lemon

- ❖ Mix well and drizzle with olive oil, coconut milk and lemon juice.
- ❖ Enjoy!

62) Almonds with sautéed vegetables

Preparation time: **Cooking time:** **Servings: 4**

Ingredients:

- ✓ Young beans, 150g
- ✓ Broccoli flower, 4
- ✓ Oregano and cumin, ½ teaspoon
- ✓ Lemon juice (fresh), 3 tablespoons
- ✓ Garlic clove (finely chopped), 1

Directions:

- ❖ Add broccoli, beans and other vegetables to a large skillet and fry until beans and broccoli turn dark green.
- ❖ Make sure the vegetables are crispy as well.
- ❖ Now add the chopped garlic and onion, sauté and stir for a few minutes.

Ingredients:

- ✓ Cauliflower, 1 cup
- ✓ Olive oil (cold pressed), 4 tablespoons
- ✓ Pepper and salt to taste
- ✓ Some soaked almonds (sliced), for garnish
- ✓ Yellow onion, 1
- ❖ Then, put the dressing together.
- ❖ Take a small bowl, add the lemon juice, oregano, cumin and oil and mix well.
- ❖ Add some vegetables, stir slowly and taste for pepper and salt.
- ❖ Finally, use the sliced almonds for garnish.
- ❖ Serve.

63) Alkaline Sweet Potato Mash

Preparation time: **Cooking time:** **Servings: 3-4**

Ingredients:

- ✓ Sea salt, 1 tablespoon
- ✓ Curry powder, ½ tablespoon
- ✓ Sweet potatoes (large), 6

Directions:

- ❖ First, get a large mixing bowl.
- ❖ Wash and cut the sweet potatoes and add them to the cooking pot and cook for about twenty minutes.

Ingredients:

- ✓ Coconut milk (fresh), 1 ½ - 2 cups
- ✓ Extra virgin olive oil (cold pressed), 1 tablespoon
- ✓ Pepper, 1 pinch

- ❖ Then, remove the sweet potatoes and mash them to your desired consistency.
- ❖ Finally, all you have to do is add the remaining ingredients and serve.

64) Mediterranean peppers

Preparation time: **Cooking time:** **Servings: 2**

Ingredients:

- ✓ Oregano, 1 teaspoon
- ✓ Garlic cloves (crushed), 2
- ✓ Fresh parsley (chopped), 2 tablespoons
- ✓ Vegetable broth (no yeast), 1 cup
- ✓ Provincial herbs, 1 teaspoon

Directions:

- ❖ Heat the olive oil in a skillet over medium heat, add the bell bell pepper and onions and stir.
- ❖ Add the garlic and stir.

Ingredients:

- ✓ Red bell pepper (sliced) 2 + Yellow bell pepper (sliced) 2
- ✓ Red onions (thinly sliced), 2 medium-sized
- ✓ Extra virgin olive oil (cold pressed), 2 tablespoons
- ✓ Salt and pepper to taste

- ❖ Then, add the vegetable stock and season with parsley and herbs, as well as pepper and salt to taste.
- ❖ Cover the pan and let it cook for fourteen to fifteen minutes.
- ❖ Serve.

65) Tomato and avocado sauce with potatoes

Preparation time: **Cooking time:**   **Servings: 3**

Ingredients:

- ✓ Red onion 1
- ✓ 2 Tomatoes
- ✓ ½ - 1 lemon (squeezed)
- ✓ Chives (fresh and chopped), 1 teaspoon
- ✓ Parsley (fresh and chopped), 1 teaspoon

Directions:

- ❖ Take a pan and cook the potatoes in salted water, (cook the potatoes with the skin intact).
- ❖ Next, peel the avocado, toss it in a bowl and mash it with a fork.

Ingredients:

- ✓ Cayenne pepper, ½ teaspoon
- ✓ Avocado (ripe), 2
- ✓ Waxy potatoes (medium size), 6
- ✓ Saltwater
- ✓ Pepper and salt
- ❖ Now, dice the onion and tomatoes, add them to the bowl along with the parsley, chives and cayenne.
- ❖ Mix well and season with pepper, lemon juice and salt.
- ❖ Serve along with the potatoes.

66) Alkaline beans and coconut

Preparation time: **Cooking time:**   **Servings: 4**

Ingredients:

- ✓ Ground cumin, ½ teaspoon
- ✓ Red chili pepper (chopped), 1-2
- ✓ Coconut milk (fresh), 3 tablespoons
- ✓ Dry flaked coconut, 1 tablespoon
- ✓ Garlic (chopped), 2 cloves
- ✓ Cayenne pepper, 1 pinch

Directions:

- ❖ Heat the oil in a skillet and add the beans, cumin, garlic, ginger and glaze and sauté for about six minutes.

Ingredients:

- ✓ Sea salt, 1 pinch
- ✓ Extra virgin olive oil (cold pressed), 3 tablespoons
- ✓ Fresh herbs of your choice, 1 teaspoon
- ✓ One (1) pound of green beans, cut into 1-inch pieces
- ✓ Fresh ginger (chopped), ½ teaspoon
- ❖ Add the coconut flakes and oil and sauté until the milk is fully cooked (this may take three or four minutes).
- ❖ Season with pepper, salt and herbs to taste. Serve.

67) Alkalized vegetable lasagna

Preparation time: **Cooking time:**   **Servings: 1**

Ingredients:

- ✓ Parsley root, 1
- ✓ Leek (small), 1
- ✓ Radish (small), 1
- ✓ Corn salad, 1
- ✓ Tomatoes (large), 3
- ✓ Garlic, 1 clove

Directions:

- ❖ Take a blender and add the lemon juice, garlic clove and avocado.
- ❖ Cut the bell bell pepper into thin strips, cut the leek into thin rings and finely grate the parsley root and radish. When you are done, mix everything with the avocado cream.

Ingredients:

- ✓ Avocado (soft), 2
- ✓ Lemon (squeezed), 1-2
- ✓ Arugula, 1
- ✓ Parsley (few)
- ✓ Red bell pepper, 1
- ❖ Let's start with the first layer of the lasagna.
- ❖ Deposit corn salad in a casserole dish, add avocado spread well.
- ❖ For the second layer, add the sliced tomatoes.
- ❖ Finally, add the arugula and parsley for the final layer.
- ❖ Serve.

68) Aloo Gobi

Preparation time: **Cooking time:**   **Servings: 1 bowl**

Ingredients:
- ✓ Cauliflower, 750g
- ✓ Fresh ginger, 20g
- ✓ Large onions, 2
- ✓ Mint, 1/3 cup
- ✓ Turmeric, 2 teaspoons
- ✓ Diced tomatoes, 400g
- ✓ Fresh garlic, 2 cloves
- ✓ Cayenne pepper, 2 teaspoons

Directions:
- ❖ Blend the chili, garlic and ginger.
- ❖ Fry oil in a wok for three minutes and add onion until golden brown.
- ❖ Add ground pasta and sauté for a few seconds, then add; garam masala, chili, turmeric, tomatoes and salt.

Ingredients:
- ✓ Cilantro/coriander leaves, 1/3 cup
- ✓ Large potatoes, 4
- ✓ Garam masala, 2 teaspoons
- ✓ Green chilli, 4
- ✓ Water, 3 cups
- ✓ Extra virgin olive oil (cold pressed), 125 ml
- ✓ Salt to taste

- ❖ Cook for about five minutes and add all other ingredients.
- ❖ Stir for three minutes and add the water.
- ❖ Cook until sauce is thick.
- ❖ Serve with Basmati rice or as a side dish.

69) Chocolate Crunch Bars

Preparation time: 3 hours   **Cooking time:** 5 minutes   **Servings: 4**

Ingredients:
- ✓ 1 1/2 cups sugar-free chocolate chips
- ✓ 1 cup of nut butter
- ✓ Stevia for taste

Directions:
- ❖ Prepare an 8-inch baking dish with baking paper.
- ❖ Mix chips chocolate with butter, coconut oil and sweetener in a bowl.
- ❖ Melt in the microwave for 2 to 3 minutes until melted.

316 Fat: 30.9g. Carbs: 8.3g. Protein: 6.4g. Fiber: 3.8g.

Ingredients:
- ✓ 1/4 cup of coconut oil
- ✓ 3 cups pecans, chopped

- ❖ Add the nut and nuts. Stir gently.
- ❖ Put this wand in the oven and then it won't open anymore.
- ❖ Refrigerate for 2 to 3 hours.
- ❖ Slice and serve.

70) Nut Butter Bars

Preparation time: 40 minutes.   **Cooking time:** 10 minutes.   **Servings: 6**

Ingredients:
- ✓ 3/4 cup of walnut flour
- ✓ 2 ounces of nut butter
- ✓ 1/4 cup Swerve

Directions:
- ❖ Combine all the ingredients for best results.
- ❖ Transfer contents to a small 6-inch baking dish. Press down firmly.

214 Fat: 19g. Carbs: 6.5g. Protein: 6.5g. Fiber: 2.1g.

Ingredients:
- ✓ 1/2 wooden walnut
- ✓ 1/2 teaspoon vanilla

- ❖ Refrigerate for 30 minutes.
- ❖ Cut into slices and serve.

71) Homemade Protein Bar

Preparation time: 5 mnutes   **Cooking time:** 10 minutes   **Servings: 4**

Ingredients:
- ✓ 1 knob of butter
- ✓ 4 tablespoons of coconut oil
- ✓ 2 scoops of vanilla protein

Directions:
- ❖ Mix coconut oil with butter, protein, stevia and salt in a dish.
- ❖ Mix cinnamon and chocolate chips.

179 Fat: 15.7g. Carbohydrates: 4.8g. Protein: 5.6g. Fiber: 0.8g.

Ingredients:
- ✓ To taste, ½ teaspoon of sea salt Optional Ingredients:
- ✓ 1 teaspoon cinnamon

- ❖ Presss the dough is firmly and freeze until firmed.
- ❖ Cut the crust into small bars.
- ❖ Serve and enjoy.

72) Shortbread Coookies

Preparation time: 10 minutes   **Cooking time**: 1 hour and 10 minutes   **Servings: 6**

Ingredients:
- ✓ 2 1/2 cups coconut flour
- ✓ 6 tablespoons of nut butter

Directions:
- ❖ Preheat our oven to 350 degrees.
- ❖ Place on a cookie sheet with the parchment paper.
- ❖ Beat the butter with the erythritol until fluffy.
- ❖ Add the vanilla essence and coconut flour.

288 Fat: 25.3g. Carbohydrates: 9.6g. Protein: 7.6g. Fiber: 3.8g.

Ingredients:
- ✓ 1/2 cup erythritol
- ✓ 1 teaspoon of vanilla essence

- ❖ Mix everything together until crumbly.
- ❖ Spoon out a tablespoon of cookie dough onto the cookie sheet.
- ❖ Add more dough to make a stack.
- ❖ Bake for 15 minutes until golden brown.
- ❖ Serve.

73) Coconut cookies Chip

Preparation time: 10 minutes   **Cooking time**: 15 minutes   **Servings: 4**

Ingredients:
- ✓ 1 cup of walnut flour
- ✓ ½ cup cacao nibs
- ✓ ½ cup coconut flakes, unsweetened
- ✓ 1/3 cup erythritol
- ✓ ½ cup nut butter

Directions:
- ❖ Prepare the oven for 350 degrees F.
- ❖ Layer a cookie sheet with parchment paper.
- ❖ Add and combine all ingredients dry in a glass bowl.
- ❖ Coconut milk, coconut milk, vanilla, stevia and peanut butter.
- ❖ Beating well compared to stir in the battery. Mix well.

192 Fat: 17.44g. Carbohydrates: 2.2g. Protein: 4.7g. Fiber: 2.1g.

Ingredients:
- ✓ ¼ cup peanut launcher, more than once
- ✓ ¼ cup of coconut milk
- ✓ Stevia, to taste
- ✓ ¼ teaspoon of sea salt

- ❖ Spoon out a tablespoon of cookie dough on the coookie shet.
- ❖ Add more dough to make 16 coookies.
- ❖ Fluctuate each cookie using your fingers.
- ❖ Water for 25 minutes until dawn.
- ❖ Let them rest for 15 minutes.
- ❖ Serve.

74) Coconut Cookies

Preparation time: 10 mnutes   **Cooking time**: 20 minutes   **Servings: 6**

Ingredients:
- ✓ 6 tablespoons coconut flour
- ✓ ¾ teaspoons baking powder
- ✓ 1/8 teaspoon sea salt
- ✓ 3 tablespoons of nut butter

Directions:
- ❖ Preheat our oven to 375 degrees F. Layer a cookie sheet with parchment.
- ❖ Place all wet ingredients in a blender. Blend all the mixture in a blender.
- ❖ Add the wet mixture and mix well until used up.

151 Fat: 13.4g. Carbs: 6.4g. Protein: 4.2g. Fiber: 4.8g

Ingredients:
- ✓ 1/6 cup coconut oil
- ✓ 6 tablespoon data sugar
- ✓ 1/3 cup coco nut milk
- ✓ 1/2 teaspoon vanilla essence
- ❖ Place a spoonful of dough cookie on the cookie sheet.
- ❖ Add a little more butter to make many coookies. Bake until golden brown (about 10 minutes). We'll see.

75) Berry Mousse

Preparation time: 5 minutes   **Cooking time:** 5 minutes   **Servings: 2**

Ingredients:

- ✓ 1 teaspoon Seville orange zest
- ✓ 3 oz. raspberries or blueberries.

Directions:

- ❖ Blend the rice in an electric blender until the fluff is dissolved.
- ❖ Add the vanilla and Seville zest. Stir well.
- ❖ Add the walnuts and berries.

265 Fat: 13g. Carbohydrates: 7.5g. Protein: 5.2g. Fiber: 0.5g.

Ingredients:

- ✓ ¼ teaspoon vanilla essence
- ✓ 2 cups coconut cream

- ❖ Cover the glove with a plastic wrench.
- ❖ Refrigerate for 3 hours.
- ❖ Garnish as desired. Serve.

76) Coconut pulp Cooookies

Preparation time: 5 minutes.   **Cooking time:** 10 hours.   **Servings: 4**

Ingredients:

- ✓ 3 cups coconut pulp
- ✓ 1 Granny Smith apple
- ✓ 1-2 teaspoon cinnamon

Directions:

- ❖ Blend the coconut with the remaining ingredients in a processor food processor.
- ❖ Make many cookies with this mixture.
- ❖ Arrange them on a kitchen table, lined with parchment.

240 Fat: 22.5g. Carbohydrates: 17.3g. Protein: 14.9g. Fiber: 0g.

Ingredients:

- ✓ 2-3 tablespoons of raw honey
- ✓ 1/4 cup coco walnut flakes

- ❖ Place the dough in a food grade oven for 6-10 hours at 115 degrees Fahrenheit.
- ❖ Serve.

77) Avocado Pudding

Preparation time: 10 minutes   **Cooking time:** 0 minutes   **Servings: 2**

Ingredients:

- ✓ 2 avocados
- ✓ 3/4-1 cup coconut milk
- ✓ 1/3-1 1/2 cup of raw cacao powder

Directions:

- ❖ Mix all ingredients together in a blender.

609 Fats: 50.5g. Carbs: 9.9g. Protein: 29.3g. Fiber: 1.5g.

Ingredients:

- ✓ 1 teaspoon 100% pure organic vanilla (optional)
- ✓ 2-4 tablespoons of date sugar

- ❖ Refrigerate for 4 hours in a container.
- ❖ Serve.

78) Coconut Raisins cooookies

Preparation time: 10 minutes.   **Cooking time:** 10 minutes.   **Servings: 4**

Ingredients:

- ✓ 1 1/4 cups of coconut flour 1 cup of nut flour
- ✓ 1 teaspoon baking soda
- ✓ 1/2 Celtic teaspoon sea salt
- ✓ 1 button for peanuts cup
- ✓ 1 cup coconut date sugar

Directions:

- ❖ Turn on the oven to 357 degrees F.
- ❖ Mix the flour with the salt and baking soda.
- ❖ Flatten with sugar until started and then stirs in the nut milk and vinavilla.

237 Fat: 19.8g. Carbs: 55.1g. Protein: 17.8g. Fiber: 0.9g.

Ingredients:

- ✓ 2 teaspoons of vanilla
- ✓ ¼ cup coconut milk
- ✓ 3/4 cup organic raisins
- ✓ 3/4 cup coconut chips or flakes

- ❖ Mix well, then place in a powder container. Stir until fine.
- ❖ Add all remaining ingredients.
- ❖ Make small cooookies out this dough.
- ❖ Arrange the cookies on a baking sheet.
- ❖ Bake for 10 minutes until set.

79) Cracker Pumpkin Spice

Preparation time: 10 minutes. **Cooking time:** 1 hour. **Servings: 6**

Ingredients:

- ✓ 1/3 cup coco walnut flour
- ✓ 2 tablespoons pumpkin pie spice
- ✓ ¾ cup sunflower seds
- ✓ ¾ cup flaxseed
- ✓ 1/3 cup sesame seeds

Ingredients:

- ✓ 1 tablespoon gron psyllium husk powder
- ✓ 1 teaspoon sea salt
- ✓ 3 tablespoons coco walnut oil, melted
- ✓ 11/3 cups water

Directions:

- ❖ Heat our oven to 300 degrees F. Combine all ingredients in a bowl.
- ❖ Add the salt and oil to the mixture and mix well.
- ❖ Allow the dough to rest for 2 to 3 minutes.

- ❖ Roll out the dough on a cookie sheet lined with parchment paper.
- ❖ Bake for 30 minutes.
- ❖ Reduce the amount of food to 30 m weight and let it rest for another 30 m.
- ❖ Crush the bread into small pieces. Serve

248 Fat: 15.7g. Carbs: 0.4g. Protein: 24.9g. Fiber: 0g.

80) Spicy Toasted nuts

Preparation time: 10 minutes. **Cooking time:** 15 minutes. **Servings: 4**

Ingredients:

- ✓ 8 ounces of pecans or coconuts or walnuts
- ✓ 1 teaspoon of sea salt
- ✓ 1 tablespoon olive oil or coconut oil

Ingredients:

- ✓ 1 teaspoon of ground cumin
- ✓ 1 teaspoon of paprika powder or chili powder

Directions:

- ❖ Add all ingredients to an oven. Brown nuts until golden brown.

- ❖ Serve and enjoy.

287 Fat: 29.5g. Carbohydrates: 5.9g. Protein: 4.2g. Fiber: 4.3g.

81) Cracker Healthy

Preparation time: **Cooking time:** 30 minutes   **Servings: 50 Crackers**

Ingredients:

- ✓ 1/2 cup of rye flour
- ✓ 1 cup of flour Spelt
- ✓ 2 teaspoons of Sesame Seed
- ✓ 1 teaspoon of Agave Syrup

Ingredients:

- ✓ 1 teaspoon of Pure Sea Salt
- ✓ 2 tablespoons of Grape Seed Oil
- ✓ 3/4 cup of Spring Water

Directions:

- ❖ Preheat our oven to 350 degrees Fahrenheit.
- ❖ Add all ingredients to a glass container and mix everything together.
- ❖ Make a ball of dough. If the dough is too thick, add more flour.
- ❖ Prepare a place to spread the dough and cover it with a piece of parchment paper.
- ❖ Degrease the container well with Grape Seed Oil and put the dart in it.
- ❖ RICE the slurry with a rolling pin, adding more flour so it doesn't fall apart.

- ❖ When your dough is ready, take a pastry cutter and insert it into the container. If you don't have a pastry cutter, you can use a cookie cutter.
- ❖ Arrange the squares on a kitchen basket and place them in the corner of a ech square using a fork of a skewer.
- ❖ Brush the plate with a little grain oil and sprinkle with a little pure sea salt, if needed.
- ❖ Bake for 12-15 minutes or until crackers are golden brown.
- ❖ Everything that was done was done with the help of another person.
- ❖ Serve and enjoy your Healthy Crackers!

82) Tortillas

Preparation time:.   **Cooking Time:** 20 Minutes   **Servings: 8**

Ingredients:

- ✓ 2 cups of flour Spelt
- ✓ 1 teaspoon of Pure Sea Salt

Ingredients:

- ✓ 1/2 cup of spring Water

Directions:

- ❖ In a food processor* blend the spelt flour with the pure salt. Blend for about 15 minutes.
- ❖ Blend, slowly add Grape seed oil until well distributed.
- ❖ Slowly add the soy water, stirring until a color forms.
- ❖ Prepare a piece of wallpaper and pour some parchment paper on it. Dust with a little flour.

- ❖ Process the nut for about 1 to 2 minutes until it reaches the right consistency.
- ❖ Pour dough into 8-inch pieces.
- ❖ Roll the sandwich into a very thin shape.
- ❖ Prepare a lunch box, cook one tortilla at a time in the microwave for about 30-60 minutes.
- ❖ Serve and enjoy your Tortillas!

83) Walnut cheesecake Mango

Preparation time: **Cooking time:** 4 hours and 30 minutes   **Servings: 8**

Ingredients:

- ✓ 2 cups of Brazil Nuts
- ✓ 5 to 6 Dates
- ✓ 1 tablespoon of Sea Moss Gel (check information)
- ✓ 1/4 cup o of agave syrup
- ✓ 1/4 teaspoon salt Pure Sea
- ✓ 2 tablespoons of Lime Juice
- ✓ 1 1/2 cups of Homemade Walnut Milk *

Ingredients:

Crust:
- ✓ 1 1/2 cups of quartered Dates 1/4 cup of Agave Syrup
- ✓ 1 1/2 cups of Coconut Flakes
- ✓ 1/4 teaspoon of Pure Sea Salt
- ✓ Toppings:
- ✓ Mango of Sliced
- ✓ Sliced strawberries
- ❖ Place the filling on top of the butter, wrap it with aluminum foil or a food container and let it rest for 3 to 4 hours in the refrigerator.
- ❖ Take out dalla baking form and garnish with toppings.
- ❖ Serve and enjoy our Mango Nut Cheesecake!

Directions:

- ❖ Place all crust ingredients in a processor and blend for 30 seconds.
- ❖ Prepare a baking sheet with a sheet of parchment and roll out the loose dough with butter.
- ❖ Place the Mango sliced across the crust and freeze for 10 minutes.
- ❖ Place all the glass pieces in a bowl until ready.

84) Blackberry Jam

Preparation time:

Cooking time: 4 hours and 30 minutes

Servings: 1 cup

Ingredients:
- ✓ 3/4 cup of Blackberries
- ✓ 1 tablespoon lime juice Key

Ingredients:
- ✓ 3 tablespoons of Agave Syrup
- ✓ ¼ cup of Sea Moss Gel + extra 2 tablespoons (check information)

❖ Add Sea Moss Gel, Key Lime Juice and Agave Syrup to the mixture. Cook over low heat and stir well until dry.
❖ Remove from heat and let sit for 10 minutes.
❖ Serve with pieces on flat bread.
❖ Enjoy your jam!

Directions:
❖ Place blackberries in a medium saucepan and cook over low heat.
❖ Stir in blackberries until liquid is gone.
❖ Once you've picked the berries, use your blender to chop up the larger pieces. If you don't have a blender, put the mixture in an immersion blender, blend it well, and then return it to the oven.

85) Blackberry Bars

Preparation time:

Cooking time: 1 hour 20 Minutes

Servings: 4

Ingredients:
- ✓ 3 Burro Banas or 4 Baby Banas
- ✓ 1 cup of Spelt Flour
- ✓ 2 cups of Quinoa Flakes
- ✓ 1/4 cup of Agave Syrup

Ingredients:
- ✓ 1/4 teaspoon of Pure Sea Salt
- ✓ 1/2 cup of Grape Seed Oil
- ✓ 1 cup of prepared Blackberry Jam

❖ Spread Blackberry Jam over the dough.
❖ Crumble the rice and place it on the plate.
❖ Bake for 20 minutes.
❖ Remove from oven and let cool for 10-15 minutes.
❖ Cut into small pieces.
❖ Try and enjoy our Blackberry Bars!

Directions:
❖ Set the oven to 350 degrees Fahrenheit.
❖ Mash the bananas with a fork in a large bowl.
❖ Combine Agave Syrup and Grape Seed Oil to the puree and mix well.
❖ Add the Spelt flour and Quinoa flakes. Knead the dough until it becomes sticky to your finger.
❖ Prepare a 9x9-inch basket with a parchment lid.
❖ Take 2/3 of the dough and spread it with your fingers on the baking sheet parchment pan.

Helpful Hints: You can store this Blackberry Bar in the refrigerator for 5-6 days or in the freezer for up to 3 months.

86) Squash Pie.

Preparation time:

Cooking time: 2 hours 30 Minutes

Servings: 6-8

Ingredients:
- ✓ 2 Butternut Squashes
- ✓ 1 1/4 cups of spelt flour
- ✓ 1/4 cup of dry sugar
- ✓ 1/4 cup of Agave Syrup
- ✓ 1 teaspoon of Allspice.

Ingredients:
- ✓ 1 teaspoon of Pure Sea Salt
- ✓ 1/4 cup soy water
- ✓ 1/3 cup of fat seed oil
- ✓ 1/4 cup hemp seed milk Homemade *

❖ Reduce the rice into a loaf of bread. Add more water or flour if needed. Let stand for 5 minutes.
❖ Spread out Spelt Flour on a piece of parchment paper.
❖ Roll out on rolling pin, adding more flour to prevent sticking.
❖ Place the dough in a cake pan and bake for 10 minutes.
❖ Remove the butter from the oven, add the filling and bake for another 40 minutes.
❖ Remove the cake and let it rest for 30 minutes until cool.
❖ Serve enjoy your Squash Pie!

Directions:
❖ Rinse and peel butternut pumpkins.
❖ Cut them in half and use a spoon to de-sed.
❖ Cut the meat into one piece and place in a glass container.
❖ Cover the squash in Spring Water and boiltare for 20-25 minutes until coooked.
❖ Turn off the oven and mash the cooked squash.
❖ Add the date sugar, agave syrup, 1/8 pure sea salt, and homemade milk and mix everything together.
❖ Crust:
❖ Preheat the oven to 350 degrees Fahrenheit.
❖ In a bowl, add the spelt flour, 1/2 teaspoon of Pure Sea Salt, Spring Water, and Grape Sed Oil and mix.

87) Walnut Milk homemade

Preparation time:

Cooking time: minimum 8 hours   **Servings: 4 cups**

Ingredients:
- ✓ 1 cup fresh walnuts
- ✓ 1/8 teaspoon of Pure Sea Salt

Ingredients:
- ✓ 3 cups of spring water + extra for soaking

Directions:
- ❖ Place the new Walnuts in a bag and fill it with three tablespoons of water.
- ❖ Take the Walnuts for an hour and a half.
- ❖ Drain and rinse nuts with warm water.

- ❖ Add the soaked walnuts, puree and three times the spring water to a blender.
- ❖ Mix well till smooth.
- ❖ Extend it if you need to.
- ❖ Enjoy your homemade nut milk!

88) Aquafaba

Preparation time:

Cooking time: 2 Hours 30 minutes   **Servings: 2-4 cups**

Ingredients:
- ✓ 1 bag of Garbanzo beans
- ✓ 1 teaspoon of Pure Sea Salt

Ingredients:
- ✓ 6 cups of Spring Water + extra for soaking

Directions:
- ❖ Place the chickpeas in a large pot, add the soy water and pure sea salt. Bring to a boil.
- ❖ Remove from heat and allow to soak 30 to 40 minutes.
- ❖ Strain the Garbanzo Beans and add 6 cups of water.
- ❖ Boil for 1 hour and 30 minutes on medium hat.

- ❖ Filter the Garbanzo beans. This filtered water is Aquafaba.
- ❖ Pour the Aquafaba into a glass jar with a lid and place in the refrigerator.
- ❖ After cooling, the Aquafaba becomes thicker. If it is too thick, boil for 10-20 mnutes.

89) Milk Homemade Hempsed

Preparation time:

Cooking time: 2 hours   **Servings: 2 cups**

Ingredients:
- ✓ 2 tablespoons of Hemp Seeds
- ✓ 2 tablespoons of Agave Syrup

Ingredients:
- ✓ 1/8 teaspoon pure salt
- ✓ 2 cups of Spring Water Fruits (optional)*.

- ❖ Store milk in the refrigerator until aged.
- ❖ Enjoy your Homemade Hempsed Milk!

Directions:
- ❖ Place all ingredients, except fruit, in blender.
- ❖ Blend them for two minutes.
- ❖ Add fruits and resin for 30-50 minutes.

90) Oil spicy infusion

Preparation time:

Cooking time: 24 Hours   **Servings: 1 cup**

Ingredients:

✓ *1 tablespoon of crushed Cayenne Pepper*

Ingredients:
- ✓ 3/4 cup of Grape Seed Oil

Directions:
- ❖ Fill a glass with a lid or bottle with grape oil.
- ❖ Add crushed Cayenne Pepper to the jar/bottle.

- ❖ Close and allow to cool for at least 24 hours.
- ❖ Add it to a dinner party and enjoy our Spicy Infuse oil!

91) Italian infused oil

Preparation time:

Cooking time: 24 hours

Servings: 1 cup

Ingredients:
- ✓ 1 teaspoon of Oregano.
- ✓ 1 teaspoon of Basil

Ingredients:
- ✓ 1 pinch of salt Pure Sea
- ✓ 3/4 cup of Grape seed oil

Directions:
- ❖ Fill a glass jar with a lid or container with grape oil.
- ❖ Mix the seasonings and add them to the rice and lettuce.

- ❖ Shake and let the oil steep for at least 24 hours.
- ❖ Add it to a dish and enjoy your Infused Oil Italian!

Helpful Hints:

92) Garlic Infused Oil

Preparation time:

Cooking time: 24 hours

Servings: 1 cup

Ingredients:
- ✓ 1/2 teaspoon of Dill
- ✓ 1/2 teaspoon of Ginger Powder
- ✓ 1 tablespoon of Onion Powder.

Ingredients:
- ✓ 1/2 teaspoon of Pure Sea Salt
- ✓ 3/4 cup of fat seed oil

Directions:
- ❖ Fill a glass jar or squeeze bottle with grapeseed oil.
- ❖ Add the seasonings to the jar/bottle.

- ❖ Close and let oil infuse for at least 24 hours.
- ❖ Add it to a dish and add your "Garlic". Infused Oil!

Helpful Hints:

93) Papaya Seeds Mango Dressing

Preparation time:

Cooking time: 10 minutes

Servings: 1/2 Cup

Ingredients:
- ✓ 1 cup of chopped Mango
- ✓ 1 teaspoon of Papaya Seeds Ground
- ✓ 1 teaspoon of Basil
- ✓ 1 teaspoon of Onion Powder

Ingredients:
- ✓ 1 teaspoon of Agave Syrup
- ✓ 2 tablespoons of lemon juice
- ✓ 1/4 cup of grape oil
- ✓ 1/4 teaspoon salt Pure Sea
- ❖ Add it to a dish and enjoy our Papaya Seed Mango Dress5ng!

Directions:
- ❖ Prepare and place all ingredients into the mixture.
- ❖ Blend for one minute until smoth.

Helpful Hints:

94) Blueberry Smoothie

Preparation time: 10 minutes

Cooking time:

Servings: 2

Ingredients:
- ✓ 2 cups of frozen blueberries
- ✓ 1 small banana

Ingredients:
- ✓ 1½ cups unsweetened almond milk
- ✓ ¼ cup ice cubes
- ❖ Pour the smoothie into two glasses and serve immediately.

Directions:
- ❖ Place all ingredients in a high speed blender and pulse until creamy.

95) Raspberry and tofu smoothie

Preparation time: 10 minutes   **Cooking time**:   **Servings: 2**

Ingredients:

✓   1½ cups of fresh raspberries
✓   6 ounces of firm silken tofu, pressed and drained
✓   4-5 drops of liquid stevia

Directions:

❖   Place all ingredients in a high speed blender and pulse until creamy.

Ingredients:

✓   1 cup of coconut cream
✓   ¼ cup ice, crushed

❖   Pour the smoothie into two glasses and serve immediately.

Helpful Hints:

96) Beet and Strawberry Smoothie

Preparation time: 10 minutes   **Cooking time**:   **Servings: 2**

Ingredients:

✓   2 cups frozen strawberries, pitted and chopped
✓   ⅔ cup roasted and frozen beet, chopped
✓   1 teaspoon fresh ginger, peeled and grated

Directions:

❖   Place all ingredients in a high speed blender and pulse until creamy.

Ingredients:

✓   1 teaspoon fresh turmeric, peeled and grated
✓   ½ cup of fresh orange juice
✓   1 cup unsweetened almond milk

❖   Pour the smoothie into two glasses and serve immediately.

97) Kiwi Smoothie

Preparation time: 10 minutes   **Cooking time**:   **Servings: 2**

Ingredients:

✓   4 kiwis
✓   2 small bananas, peeled
✓   1½ cups unsweetened almond milk

Directions:

❖   Place all ingredients in a high speed blender and pulse until creamy.

Ingredients:

✓   1-2 drops of liquid stevia
✓   ¼ cup ice cubes

❖   Pour the smoothie into two glasses and serve immediately.

98) Pineapple and Carrot Smoothie

Preparation time: 10 minutes   **Cooking time**:   **Servings: 2**

Ingredients:

✓   1 cup frozen pineapple
✓   1 large ripe banana, peeled and sliced
✓   ½ tablespoon fresh ginger, peeled and chopped
✓   ¼ teaspoon ground turmeric

Directions:

❖   Place all ingredients in a high speed blender and pulse until creamy.

Ingredients:

✓   1 cup unsweetened almond milk
✓   ½ cup fresh carrot juice
✓   1 tablespoon fresh lemon juice

❖   Pour the smoothie into two glasses and serve immediately.

99) Oatmeal and orange smoothie

Preparation time: 10 minutes   **Cooking time**:   **Servings: 4**

Ingredients:

✓   ⅔ cup of rolled oats
✓   2 oranges, peeled, seeds removed and cut into sections
✓   2 large bananas, peeled and sliced

Directions:

❖   Place all ingredients in a high speed blender and pulse until creamy.

Ingredients:

✓   2 cups of unsweetened almond milk
✓   1 cup ice cubes, crushed

❖   Pour the smoothie into four glasses and serve immediately.

100) *Pumpkin Smoothie*

Preparation time: 10 minutes

Cooking time:

Servings: 2

Ingredients:

- ✓ 1 cup homemade pumpkin puree
- ✓ 1 medium banana, peeled and sliced
- ✓ 1 tablespoon maple syrup
- ✓ 1 teaspoon ground flax seeds

Directions:

- ❖ Place all ingredients in a high speed blender and pulse until creamy.

Ingredients:

- ✓ ½ teaspoon ground cinnamon
- ✓ ¼ teaspoon ground ginger
- ✓ 1½ cups unsweetened almond milk
- ✓ ¼ cup ice cubes
- ❖ Pour the smoothie into two glasses and serve immediately.

Chapter 7 -   Dr. Lewis's Meal Plan Project

Day 1

1) Blueberry Muffins

23) Vegetable and berry salad

41) Mixed stew of spicy vegetables

64) Mediterranean peppers

86) Squash Pie.

Day 2

4) "Chocolate" Pudding.

25) Grab and Go Wraps

46) Curried red beans

61) Quinoa Salad

100) Pumpkin Smoothie

Day 3

7) Strawberry and Beet Smoothie

28) Avocado and salmon soup

51) Quinoa with vegetables

67) Alkalized vegetable lasagna

87) Walnut Milk homemade

Day 4

11) Orange and Oat Smoothie

31) Spicy cabbage bowl

55) Chickpeas with pumpkin

73) Coconut cookies Chip

99) Oatmeal and orange smoothie

Day 5

18) Pecan Pancakes

33) Vegan Burger

58) Green beans and mushrooms in casserole

71) Homemade Protein Bar

82) Tortillas

Day 6

16) Hemp seed and carrot muffins

37) Walnut, date, orange and cabbage salad

59) Meatloaf of wild rice and lentils

80) Spicy Toasted nuts

89) Milk Homemade Hempsed

Day 7

19) Quinoa Breakfast

40) Alkalizing millet dish

54) Spicy baked beans

77) Avocado Pudding

83) Walnut cheesecake Mango

Chapter 8 -   Conclusion

I hope this book can lead you to your goals, keeping your desire to keep going high, without making you lose sight of the outcome

This book series is designed to help women, men, athletes and sportsmen, people immersed in work with little free time, etc.

If you recognize yourself in one of these categories or someone you know has decided to take the same path as you,

You'll find the other books in the series in your trusted bookstore, guaranteed!

Big hugs from Dr. Grace!

Alkaline Diet Cookbook on a Budget

Dr. Lewis's Meal Plan Project| 100 Affordable, Easy-To-Prepare Recipes to Kickstart Your Long-Term Transformation Path Without Emptying Your Wallet

By Grace Lewis

Chapter 1 -   Introduction

Starting a diet path may be the hardest choice to make, but it will be the best choice you will ever make in your life.

The alkaline diet can help you embark on your path of change much more easily than other diet paths.

In most cases an individual is inclined to think that rigidly adhering to a diet plan will lead him or her to spend much more money than the family budget normally allows.

In this book I have put together all my best low budget recipes, accompanied by an eating plan to experience the benefits of the alkaline diet right away.

The important thing is to get started, without thinking about your wallet.

I wish you a speedy achievement of your goals.

Here's to your success!

Grace

Alkaline Diet Breakfast Recipes

1) Mile Porridge

Preparation time: 10 minutes.   **Cooking time:** 20 minutes.   **Servings:** 2

Ingredients:
- ✓ Sea salt
- ✓ 1 tbsp. finely chopped coconuts.
- ✓ 1/2 cup unsweetened coconut milk

Directions:
- ❖ Sauté the millet in a non-stick skillet for about 3 minutes.
- ❖ Add salt and water, then stir.
- ❖ Allow the meal to rest and reduce the amount of salt.

Nutrition: Calories

Ingredients:
- ✓ 1/2 cup millet rinsed and millet draned
- ✓ 1-1/2 cups water alkaline
- ✓ 3 Drops liquid stevia.
- ❖ Cook for about 15 minutes, then add remaining ingredients. Stylize.
- ❖ Cook the apple for an additional 4 minutes.
- ❖ Serve the meal with a garnish of hazelnuts chopped.

2) Jackfruit Fry vegetable

Preparation time: 5 minutes.   **Cooking time:** 5 minutes.   **Servings:** 6

Ingredients:
- ✓ 2 onions small finely chopped
- ✓ 2 cups tomatoes chopped cherry finely
- ✓ 1/8 tablespoon of cassava butter
- ✓ 1 tablespoon olive oil

Directions:
- ❖ In a fat skillet, saute onions and bell peppers for about 5 minutes.
- ❖ Add tomatoes and stir.
- ❖ Coook for 2 minutes.

Nutrition: Calories

Ingredients:
- ✓ 2 seeded and chopped red bell peppers
- ✓ 3 cups firm jackfruit with seeds and chopped
- ✓ 1/8 teaspoon cayenne pepper
- ✓ 2 tbsps. Chopped fresh basil leaves Salt
- ❖ Then add the juice, pepper, salt and turmeric.
- ❖ Bake for about 8 minutes.
- ❖ Garnish the meal with basil leaves.
- ❖ Serve hot.

3) Zucchini Pancakes

Preparation time: 15 minutes.   **Cooking time:** 8 minutes.   **Servings:** 8

Ingredients:
- ✓ 12 tablespoons of alkaline water
- ✓ 6 great zucchini grateds
- ✓ Sea salt
- ✓ 4 tbsp of Flax Seeds chopped

Directions:
- ❖ In a bowl, mix together the water and flax and then set aside.
- ❖ Place our food in a large non-stick container and then place it in a cooking container.
- ❖ Add the glass of milk, the glass of wine, and the glass of pumpkin.
- ❖ Coook for 3 minutes then transfer the zucchini into a large boge.

Nutrition: Calories

Ingredients:
- ✓ 2 tsps. Olive oil
- ✓ 2 jalapeño peppers finely chopped
- ✓ 1/2 cup finely chopped scallions
- ❖ Add the flax and scallion mixture and then mix everything together.
- ❖ Preheat a grill and then grease it well with oil.
- ❖ Pour 1/4 zuchini mixture into a griddle and bake for 3 minutes.
- ❖ Flip the side carefully then coook for 2 more minutes.
- ❖ Repeat the procedure with the rest of the mass in random order.
- ❖ Serve.

4) Squash Hash

Preparation time: 2 mnutes.   **Cooking time:** 10 minutes.   **Servings:** 2

Ingredients:
- ✓ 1 tsp. onion powder.
- ✓ 1/2 cup finely chopped onion

Directions:
- ❖ By using paper towels, you can get extra moisture from the spaghetti squash.
- ❖ Place the squash in a bowl, then add the salt, onion and onion powder.
- ❖ Stir well to mix everything together.
- ❖ Spray a non-stick cooking skillet with coooking spray that place il over moderate heat.

Ingredients:
- ✓ 2 cups of spaghetti squash
- ✓ 1/2 teaspoon of sea salt
- ❖ Add the spaghetti squash.
- ❖ Coook the squash for 5 minutes.
- ❖ Smash the browns with a spatula.
- ❖ Coook formatis of 5 minutes until the desired crispness is reached.
- ❖ Serve.

5) _Hemp Seed Porridge_

Preparation time: 5 minutes.

Cooking time: 5 minutes.

Servings: 6

Ingredients:
- ✓ 3 cups cooked hemp sed
- ✓ 1 packet Stevia

Ingredients:
- ✓ 1 cup coco of walnut milk

Directions:
- ❖ In a bowl, mix the milk and nut milk for about 5 minutes.
- ❖ Remove the pan from the heat and add the stevia. Stylize.

- ❖ Serve in 6 bowls.
- ❖ Enjoy.

6) _Veggie Medley_

Preparation time: 5 mnutes.

Cooking time: 10 minutes.

Servings: 2

Ingredients:
- ✓ 1 seed and 1 bacon
- ✓ 1/2 cup lime juice
- ✓ 2 tablespoons of fresh cilantro
- ✓ 1/2 tsp. cumin
- ✓ 1 teaspoon of sea salt
- ✓ 1 wooden jacket

Ingredients:
- ✓ 1/2 cup zucchini
- ✓ 1 cup halved cherry tomatoes
- ✓ 1/2 cup sliced mushrooms
- ✓ 1 cup coooked broccoli florets
- ✓ 1 sweet onion chopped

Directions:
- ❖ Spray some paint with stick pan with cooking spray and then put it all over your body.
- ❖ Add the butter, tomatoes, chili, grapes, pumpkin, peanut butter and mushroms.

- ❖ Cook for about 7 minutes as you stir from time to time.
- ❖ Add the cumin and caraway and then the pepper.
- ❖ Cook for an additional 3 minutes, stirring.
- ❖ Heat the pan off the heat and add the lime juice.
- ❖ Serve.

7) _Pumpkin Spice Quinoa_

Preparation time: 10 minutes.

Cooking time: 0 minutes.

Servings: 2

Ingredients:
- ✓ 1 cup of cooked quinoa
- ✓ 1 cup unsweetened coconut milk
- ✓ 1 large mashed banana

Ingredients:
- ✓ 1/4 cup pumpkin pureee
- ✓ 1 tsp. pumpkin spice
- ✓ 2 teaspoons of chia seds

- ❖ Refrigerate overnight.
- ❖ Serve.

Directions:
- ❖ In a container, mix all ingredients together.
- ❖ Close the lid and then close the container so that it mixes.

8) _Coconut pulp Coookies_

Preparation time: 5 minutes.

Cooking time: 10 hours.

Servings: 4

Ingredients:
- ✓ 3 cups coconut pulp
- ✓ 1 Granny Smith apple
- ✓ 1-2 teaspoon cinnamon

Ingredients:
- ✓ 2-3 tablespoons of raw honey
- ✓ 1/4 cup coco walnut flakes

Directions:
- ❖ Blend the coconut with the remaining ingredients in a processor food processor.
- ❖ Make many cookies with this mixture.
- ❖ Arrange them on a kitchen table, lined with parchment.

- ❖ Place the dough in a food grade oven for 6-10 hours at 115 degrees Fahrenheit.
- ❖ Serve.

Nutrition: Calories 240 Fat: 22.5g. Carbohydrates: 17.3g. Protein: 14.9g. Fiber: 0g.

9) _Avocado Pudding_

Preparation time: 10 minutes

Cooking time: 0 minutes

Servings: 2

Ingredients:
- ✓ 2 avocados
- ✓ 3/4-1 cup coconut milk
- ✓ 1/3-1/2 cup of raw cacao powder

Ingredients:
- ✓ 1 teaspoon 100% pure organic vanilla (optional)
- ✓ 2-4 tablespoons of date sugar

- ❖ Refrigerate for 4 hours in a container.
- ❖ Serve.

Directions:
- ❖ Mix all ingredients together in a blender.

10) Coconut Raisins cooookies

Preparation time: 10 minutes.   **Cooking time**: 10 minutes.   **Servings**: 4

Ingredients:

- ✓ 1 1/4 cups of coconut flour 1 cup of nut flour
- ✓ 1 teaspoon baking soda
- ✓ 1/2 Celtic teaspoon sea salt
- ✓ 1 button for peanuts cup
- ✓ 1 cup coconut date sugar

Directions:

- ❖ Turn on the oven to 357 degrees F.
- ❖ Mix the flour with the salt and baking soda.
- ❖ Flatten with sugar until started and then stirs in the nut milk and vinavilla.

Ingredients:

- ✓ 2 teaspoons of vanilla
- ✓ ¼ cup coconut milk
- ✓ 3/4 cup organic raisins
- ✓ 3/4 cup coconut chips or flakes

- ❖ Mix well, then place in a powder container. Stir until fine.
- ❖ Add all remaining ingredients.
- ❖ Make small cooookies out this dough.
- ❖ Arrange the cookies on a baking sheet.
- ❖ Bake for 10 minutes until set.

11) Cracker Pumpkin Spice

Preparation time: 10 minutes.   **Cooking time**: 1 hour.   **Servings**: 6

Ingredients:

- ✓ 1/3 cup coco walnut flour
- ✓ 2 tablespoons pumpkin pie spice
- ✓ ¾ cup sunflower seds
- ✓ ¾ cup flaxseed
- ✓ 1/3 cup sesame seeds

Directions:

- ❖ Heat our oven to 300 degrees F. Combine all ingredients in a bowl.
- ❖ Add the salt and oil to the mixture and mix well.
- ❖ Allow the dough to rest for 2 to 3 minutes.

Ingredients:

- ✓ 1 tablespoon gron psyllium husk powder
- ✓ 1 teaspoon sea salt
- ✓ 3 tablespoons coco walnut oil, melted
- ✓ 1 1/3 cups water

- ❖ Roll out the dough on a cookie sheet lined with parchment paper.
- ❖ Bake for 30 minutes.
- ❖ Reduce the amount of food to 30 m weight and let it rest for another 30 m.
- ❖ Crush the bread into small pieces. Serve

Nutrition: Calories 248 Fat: 15.7g. Carbs: 0.4g. Protein: 24.9g. Fiber: 0g.

12) Spicy Toasted nuts

Preparation time: 10 minutes.   **Cooking time**: 15 minutes.   **Servings**: 4

Ingredients:

- ✓ 8 ounces of pecans or coconuts or walnuts
- ✓ 1 teaspoon of sea salt
- ✓ 1 tablespoon olive oil or coconut oil

Directions:

- ❖ Add all ingredients to an oven. Brown nuts until golden brown.

Ingredients:

- ✓ 1 teaspoon of ground cumin
- ✓ 1 teaspoon of paprika powder or chili powder

- ❖ Serve and enjoy.

13) Wheat Crackers

Preparation time: 10 minutes.

Cooking time: 20 minutes.

Servings: 4

Ingredients:

- ✓ 1 3/4 cup of walnut flour
- ✓ 1 1/2 cups coconut flour
- ✓ 3/4 teaspoon sea salt

Directions:

- ❖ Set your oven to 350 degrees F.
- ❖ Mix the coconut flour, nut flour and salt in a bowl.
- ❖ Stir in vegetable oil and salt. Stir well until cooked through.
- ❖ Pour the dough onto a flat surface in a thin dish.

Ingredients:

- ✓ 1/3 vegetable oil
- ✓ 1 kitchen basket
- ✓ Sea salt for sprinkling
- ❖ Cut small squares out of the sheet.
- ❖ Arrange dough squares on a sheet of baking paper lined with parchment paper.
- ❖ Wet for 20 minutes until the light comes on.
- ❖ Serve.

14) Chips potato

Preparation time: 10 mnutes.

Cooking time: 5 minutes.

Servings: 4

Ingredients:

- • 1 tablespoon of vegetable oil

Directions:

- ❖ Toss potato with oil and sea salt.
- ❖ Distribute the slices in a sandwich dish in a single row.

Ingredients:

- ✓ 1 potato, sliced paper thin Sea salt, to taste
- ❖ Bake for 5 minutes until golden brown.
- ❖ Serve.

15) Zucchini Pepper Chips

Preparation time: 10 minutes.

Cooking time: 15 minutes.

Servings: 4

Ingredients:

- ✓ 1 2/3 cups vegetable oil
- ✓ 1 teaspoon onion powder
- ✓ 1/2 teaspoon of black pepper

Directions:

- ❖ Mix the oil with all the spices in a bowl.
- ❖ Add the zucchini slices and mix well.
- ❖ Transfer the mixture into a container Zip lock and seal il.

Ingredients:

- ✓ 3 tablespoons crushed red pepper flakes
- ✓ 2 zucchini, thinly sliced
- ❖ Refrigerate for 10 minutes.
- ❖ Spread the zuchini slices on a greased baking sheet.
- ❖ Bake for 15 minutes
- ❖ Serve.

16) Flat bread

Preparation time:

Cooking Time: 20 Minutes

Servings: 6

Ingredients:

- ✓ 2 cups of Spelt Flour
- ✓ 2 teaspoons of Oregano
- ✓ 2 teaspoons of Onion powder
- ✓ 1/4 teaspoon of Cayenne

Directions:

- ❖ Add spelt flour and all grains to a bowl and mix well.
- ❖ Add the Grape Seed Oil and 1/2 cup of Spring Water and continue to mix.
- ❖ Try to form a thick ball. If it is too thick, add more Spring Water.
- ❖ Make a place to roll the mud and sprinkle it with flour.
- ❖ Knead the dough for about 5 minutes until it has become desired consistencyn.
- ❖ Divite the dough into 6 equal balls.

Ingredients:

- ✓ 2 teaspoons of basil
- ✓ 1 tablespoon of Pure Sea Salt
- ✓ 3/4 cup o of spring water
- ✓ 2 tablespoons of Grape Seed Oil
- ❖ Roll out each loaf in a circles container about 4 inches in diameter.
- ❖ Prepare a wooden skillet. Place one flatbred in the skillet and cook over medium heat.
- ❖ Flip the dish over for 2 to 3 minutes and work until dry. Small pieces of sugar paper should be placed on both sides.
- ❖ Keep looking at the upper body.
- ❖ Serve and enjoy your Flatbread!

17) Cracker Healthy

Preparation time: **Cooking time:** 30 minutes   **Servings: 50 Crackers**

Ingredients:

- ✓ 1/2 cup of rye flour
- ✓ 1 cup of flour Spelt
- ✓ 2 teaspoons of Sesame Seed
- ✓ 1 teaspoon of Agave Syrup

Ingredients:

- ✓ 1 teaspoon of Pure Sea Salt
- ✓ 2 tablespoons of Grape Seed Oil
- ✓ 3/4 cup of Spring Water

Directions:

- ❖ Preheat our oven to 350 degrees Fahrenheit.
- ❖ Add all ingredients to a glass container and mix everything together.
- ❖ Make a ball of dough. If the dough is too thick, add more flour.
- ❖ Prepare a place to spread the dough and cover it with a piece of parchment paper.
- ❖ Degrease the container well with Grape Seed Oil and put the dart in it.
- ❖ RICE the slurry with a rolling pin, adding more flour so it doesn't fall apart.

- ❖ When your dough is ready, take a pastry cutter and insert it into the container. If you don't have a pastry cutter, you can use a cookie cutter.
- ❖ Arrange the squares on a kitchen basket and place them in the corner of a ech square using a fork of a skewer.
- ❖ Brush the plate with a little grain oil and sprinkle with a little pure sea salt, if needed.
- ❖ Bake for 12-15 minutes or until crackers are golden brown.
- ❖ Everything that was done was done with the help of another person.
- ❖ Serve and enjoy your Healthy Crackers!

Nutrition: Calories

Helpful Hints: You can add any seasonings from the Doctor Sebi's food list according to your desire. You can make crackers with our tomato sauce, avocado sauce or cheese. Sauce.

18) Tortillas

Preparation time:.   **Cooking Time:** 20 Minutes   **Servings: 8**

Ingredients:

- ✓ 2 cups of flour Spelt
- ✓ 1 teaspoon of Pure Sea Salt

Ingredients:

- ✓ 1/2 cup of spring Water

Directions:

- ❖ In a food processor* blend the spelt flour with the pure salt. Blend for about 15 minutes.
- ❖ Blend, slowly add Grape seed oil until well distributed.
- ❖ Slowly add the soy water, stirring until a color forms.
- ❖ Prepare a piece of wallpaper and pour some parchment paper on it. Dust with a little flour.

- ❖ Process the nut for about 1 to 2 minutes until it reaches the right consistency.
- ❖ Pour dough into 8-inch pieces.
- ❖ Roll the sandwich into a very thin shape.
- ❖ Prepare a lunch box, cook one tortilla at a time in the microwave for about 30-60 minutes.
- ❖ Serve and enjoy your Tortillas!

19) Pink Smoothie

Preparation time: 10 minutes   **Cooking time:** 0 minutes   **Servings: 1**

Ingredients:

- ✓ 1 peach, core and peel
- ✓ 6 ripe strawberries

Ingredients:

- ✓ 1 cup of almond milk

Directions:

- ❖ Add all ingredients to a blender.

- ❖ Blend well until smooth.
- ❖ Serve with your favorite berries

Nutrition: Calories

20) Green Apple Smoothie

Preparation time: 10 minutes   **Cooking time:** 0 minutes   **Servings: 1**

Ingredients:

- ✓ 1 peach, peeled and pitted
- ✓ 1 green apple, peeled and cored

Ingredients:

- ✓ 1 cup of alkaline water

Directions:

- ❖ Add all ingredients to a blender.

- ❖ Blend well until smooth.
- ❖ Serve with apple slices.

Alkaline Diet Lunch Recipes

21) Roasted artichoke salad

Preparation time: Cooking time: Servings: 2

Ingredients:

- ✓ Paprika, pinch
- ✓ Garlic powder, a pinch
- ✓ Pepper, pinch
- ✓ Sea salt, a pinch
- ✓ Avocado oil, 1 tablespoon
- ✓ Drained artichoke hearts, 14 ounces
- ✓ Mixed salad, 2-4 c.

Directions:

- ❖ Start by setting the oven to 425. Place parchment on a baking sheet.
- ❖ Cut off the tips of the artichokes and then cut the hearts in half. Rub them with a little oil.
- ❖ Stir in paprika, garlic, pepper and salt. Arrange artichokes on baking sheet and sprinkle with seasoning mixture. Stir to coat.

Ingredients:

- ✓ Seasoning -
- ✓ Pepper, pinch
- ✓ Sea salt, a pinch
- ✓ Shallot diced
- ✓ Brown rice sweetener, 1 tablespoon
- ✓ Sesame seeds, 1 tablespoon
- ✓ Apple vinegar, 2 tablespoons
- ✓ Avocado oil, 2 tablespoons
- ❖ Roast them for 30 minutes, tossing again halfway through the cooking time.
- ❖ While the artichokes are roasting, whisk together the pepper, salt, shallots, brown rice syrup, sesame seeds, vinegar and avocado oil. Make sure everything is well blended. Adjust the flavors as needed.
- ❖ To assemble the salad, toss the salad with the artichokes and then pour in the dressing. Divide between two plates and enjoy.

22) Artichoke pie

Preparation time: Cooking time: Servings: 4

Ingredients:

- ✓ Sliced shallot
- ✓ EVOO
- ✓ Pepper

Directions:

- ❖ Pour cold water into a bowl.
- ❖ Place the sliced artichokes in the water and let them rest.
- ❖ Rinse well and pat dry with paper towels.
- ❖ Place a skillet over medium heat and heat a little EVOO.

Nutrition: Calories

Ingredients:

- ✓ Halls
- ✓ Brussels sprouts thinly sliced, 6
- ✓ Sliced mushrooms, 4
- ❖ Add the artichokes and Brussels sprouts. Cook for four minutes.
- ❖ Sprinkle with pepper and salt.
- ❖ Serve with a drizzle of olive oil and sprinkle with sliced scallions

23) Vegetable fritters

Preparation time: Cooking time: Servings: 2

Ingredients:

- ✓ Kitchen spray
- ✓ Water, .25 c.
- ✓ Garlic powder, .5 tsp
- ✓ Salt, 1 teaspoon
- ✓ Almond flour, .25 c.

Directions:

- ❖ Place the scallions, almond flour, yellow squash, zucchini, carrot, garlic powder and salt in a food processor.
- ❖ Pulse until everything is completely mixed.
- ❖ Add just enough water to make sure the dough is moist and thick.

Ingredients:

- ✓ Shallots, 4
- ✓ Grated onion, .5
- ✓ Chopped yellow pumpkin, 1
- ✓ Peeled and chopped carrot, 1
- ✓ Chopped zucchini, 1
- ❖ Place a large skillet over standard heat and spray with prep spray.
- ❖ When the oil is heated, use an ice cream scoop and add the mixture to the pan. Cook for three minutes per side.
- ❖ Use the back of the ice cream scoop to spread the mixture.

24) Mint and lime salad

Preparation time: Cooking time: Servings: 4

Ingredients:

- ✓ Lemon juice, 2 tablespoons
- ✓ Chopped mint, 2 tablespoons
- ✓ Strawberries, .25 c.
- ✓ Diced peaches, .25 c.
- ✓ Mandarin segments, .25 c.

Directions:

- ❖ Place all the fruit in a bowl. Add the mint and lemon juice.

Nutrition: Calories

Ingredients:

- ✓ Chopped melon pieces, .25 c.
- ✓ Pieces of honeydew chunks, .25 c.
- ✓ Watermelon chunks, .25 c.
- ✓ Diced apple, .25 c.
- ✓ Grapes, .25 c.
- ❖ Mix well and cover.
- ❖ Refrigerate and chill overnight.

25) Zucchini salad

Preparation time: Cooking time: Servings: 2

Ingredients:

- ✓ Fresh herbs of your choice, 1 teaspoon
- ✓ Pepper
- ✓ Halls
- ✓ EVOO, 2 tablespoons
- ✓ Juice of 0,5 lemons

Directions:

- ❖ Wash all the vegetables and set aside.
- ❖ Cut off the ends of the zucchini. Cut in half lengthwise and then slice into half moons.
- ❖ Dice the tomatoes.
- ❖ Cut the bell bell pepper in half, clean the ribs and seeds and slice each half.

Nutrition: Calories

Ingredients:

- ✓ Chopped garlic, 1 clove
- ✓ Sliced onion, 1
- ✓ Diced tomato, 2
- ✓ Red bell pepper, 1
- ✓ Sliced zucchini, 1
- ❖ Cut off top and bottom of onion and remove outer skin. Thinly slice into rings.
- ❖ Add all prepared vegetables to a bowl.
- ❖ In a separate bowl, add pepper, salt, herbs, olive oil, garlic and lemon juice. Mix well to combine.
- ❖ Pour over vegetables and stir to coat.

26) Fried tofu

Preparation time: Cooking time: Portions:

Ingredients:

- ✓ Fresh herbs
- ✓ Ginger, .25 tablespoons
- ✓ Curry powder, .5 tablespoons
- ✓ Pepper
- ✓ Halls
- ✓ EVOO, 2 tablespoons
- ✓ Coconut milk, 1.5 c.
- ✓ Chopped green beans, .5 lb.

Directions:

- ❖ Place a saucepan over medium heat, heat the oil. Add the tofu and cook about three minutes.
- ❖ Add the zucchini, beans and peppers. Sauté for an additional three minutes.

Ingredients:

- ✓ Diced bell pepper - green, bell, 1 piece
- ✓ Diced red bell pepper, bell, 1 piece
- ✓ Diced tomatoes, 3
- ✓ Chopped zucchini, 3
- ✓ Diced firm tofu, 1 lb.

- ❖ Add the tomatoes and coconut milk and mix well. Allow to simmer for a bit longer.
- ❖ Season with herbs, curry powder, pepper, salt and ginger.
- ❖ Serve with wild rice.

27) Potato and pumpkin meatballs

Preparation time: Cooking time: Servings: 2

Ingredients:

- ✓ EVOO
- ✓ Pepper
- ✓ Halls
- ✓ Chopped parsley, 3 tablespoons

Directions:

- ❖ Peel the potatoes and squash. Cut them into large pieces.
- ❖ Place in a food processor and process until small pieces but not mush.
- ❖ Add the water and soy flour to a bowl. Stir well.
- ❖ Remove the squash and potato from the food processor and place them in another bowl.

Nutrition: Calories

Ingredients:

- ✓ Water, 4 tablespoons
- ✓ Soybean flour, 2.5 ounces
- ✓ Potatoes, 1 lb.
- ✓ Pumpkin, 1 lb.
- ❖ Pour over flour mixture and mix well.
- ❖ Season with pepper, parsley and salt.
- ❖ Place a skillet over medium heat and heat a little EVOO.
- ❖ Turn the potato and pumpkin mixture into meatballs. Place the prepared patties in the skillet and fry for three minutes per side.

28) Italian soffritto

Preparation time: Cooking time: Servings: 2

Ingredients:

- ✓ Water, .5 c
- ✓ Pepper
- ✓ Curry powder, .5 teaspoons
- ✓ Oregano plant, 1 teaspoon
- ✓ Parsley, one tablespoon
- ✓ Sodium chloride, 1 teaspoon

Directions:

- ❖ Take a frying pan and heat the olive oil.
- ❖ Place the onions in the skillet and cook until soft.
- ❖ Add the zucchini and cook an additional four minutes. Pour the water into the pan and put a lid on.
- ❖ Lower the heat and simmer for ten minutes.

Nutrition: Calories

Ingredients:

- ✓ Grated Cheddar, 1 tablespoon
- ✓ EVOO, 2 tablespoons
- ✓ Diced tomatoes, 2
- ✓ Zucchini flakes, 1
- ✓ Diced onion, 2
- ✓ Leeks in flakes, 2
- ❖ Carefully remove the lid and add the tomatoes. Season with curry powder and pepper. Replace the lid and cook another ten minutes.
- ❖ When cooked, taste and adjust seasonings if necessary.
- ❖ Sprinkle with cheese and serve with bread, if your diet permits.

29) Southern Salad

Preparation time: Cooking time: Servings: 4

Ingredients:

- ✓ Sauce, .5 c.
- ✓ Cilantro, .5 c.
- ✓ Chopped almonds, .25 c.
- ✓ Diced avocado, 1

Directions:

- ❖ Place each content in a large bowl and mix well.

Nutrition: Calories

Ingredients:

- ✓ Halved cherry tomatoes, 1 c.
- ✓ Sprouted black beans, .5 c.
- ✓ Romaine lettuce, 5 c.

- ❖ Divide among salad bowls and serve.

30) Roasted vegetables

Preparation time: Cooking time: Servings: 4

Ingredients:

- ✓ Halls
- ✓ Allium (garlic) powder, 1 tablespoon
- ✓ Coconut oil, 1 tablespoon
- ✓ Pepper - crushed, yellow bell, one
- ✓ Pepper - crushed, red bell, one

Directions:

- ❖ You need to heat the oven to 425.
- ❖ Place the carrot, peppers, tomatoes, mushrooms and asparagus in a large bowl.
- ❖ In another bowl, place the garlic powder, sodium chloride and coconut milk. Mix well.

Nutrition: Calories

Ingredients:

- ✓ Chopped carrot, one
- ✓ Cut asparagus, .5 bunch
- ✓ Cherry tomatoes, 1 pint
- ✓ Halved mushrooms, .5 c.

- ❖ Pass over the vegetables and stir to coat.
- ❖ Pour vegetables onto a cooking wrap and place on the stove for 15 minutes until vegetables are tender.
- ❖ Divide among four plates and enjoy.

31) Pad Thai Salad

Preparation time: Cooking time: Servings: 2

Ingredients:

- ✓ Salt, .5 tsp
- ✓ Stevia, 1 packet
- ✓ Tamarind paste, 1 teaspoon
- ✓ Chopped garlic, 1 clove
- ✓ Juice of a lime
- ✓ Chopped almonds, 2 tablespoons

Directions:

- ❖ Place the almonds, bean sprouts, zucchini, carrots and lettuce in a large bowl.
- ❖ Place the salt, stevia, lime juice, tamarind paste and garlic in a small food processor. Process until well blended.

Nutrition: Calories

Ingredients:

- ✓ Chopped shallot, 1
- ✓ Peeled zucchini, 1
- ✓ Thinly sliced carrot, 2
- ✓ Bean sprouts, 1 c.
- ✓ Iceberg lettuce, 4 c.

- ❖ Pour the dressing over the vegetables and toss to coat.
- ❖ Divide evenly among serving bowls.

32) Cucumber salad

Preparation time: Cooking time: Servings: 4

Ingredients:

- ✓ Pepper
- ✓ Halls
- ✓ Sesame seed oil, 3 tablespoons

Directions:

- ❖ Place the pepper, salt, sesame seed oil and garlic in a bowl. Whisk well to combine. Wash cucumbers and trim ends.

Nutrition: Calories

Ingredients:

- ✓ Chopped garlic, 4 cloves
- ✓ Cucumber, 1 lb.

- ❖ Cut them in half lengthwise and then slice them into crescents.
- ❖ Add the dressing mixture to the cucumbers and toss well to coat.
- ❖ Place in the refrigerator for ten minutes. Enjoy.

33) Pasta salad with red lentils

Preparation time:　　　　Cooking time:　　　　Servings: 4

Ingredients:

- ✓ For the dressing and pasta -
- ✓ Pepper, .25 tsp
- ✓ Sea salt, .25 tsp
- ✓ Dried oregano, 1 teaspoon
- ✓ Lemon juice, one tablespoon
- ✓ Apple vinegar, two tablespoons
- ✓ Avocado - oil, .25 c.
- ✓ Red lentil pasta, 2 c.

Directions:

- ❖ Cook pasta according to package directions.
- ❖ While the pasta is cooking, whisk together the pepper, salt, oregano, lemon juice, vinegar and avocado oil until well combined. Adjust the seasoning as needed.

Nutrition: Calories

Ingredients:

- ✓ Vegetables -
- ✓ Crushed garlic, 2 cloves
- ✓ Sliced summer squash, .5
- ✓ Sliced zucchini, .5
- ✓ Diced red onion, .33 c.
- ✓ Chopped bell pepper - orange, bell, 1 c.
- ✓ Chopped asparagus stalks, 6
- ✓ Avocado oil, 1 tablespoon
- ❖ For the vegetables, heat the oil in a large skillet and cook the garlic, squash, zucchini, onion, bell bell pepper and asparagus. Cook for two to three minutes, or until soft.
- ❖ Add pasta, vegetables and dressing to a bowl and toss. Divide among four plates and enjoy.

34) Salad with peach sauce

Preparation time:　　　　Cooking time:　　　　Servings: 2

Ingredients:

- ✓ Seasoning -
- ✓ Pinch of sea salt
- ✓ Lemon juice, 1 teaspoon
- ✓ Water, .25 c
- ✓ Brown rice syrup, 3 to 4 tablespoons
- ✓ Tahini, 4 tablespoons
- ✓ Sauce -
- ✓ Diced Jalapeno, .5

Directions:

- ❖ For the dressing, whisk together the salt, lemon juice, water, brown rice syrup and tahini until combined. Adjust seasonings as needed.

Nutrition: Calories

Ingredients:

- ✓ Chopped purple onion, one tablespoon
- ✓ Diced coriander, one tablespoon
- ✓ Chopped bell pepper - red, bell, .25 c.
- ✓ Peach cut into cubes and pitted
- ✓ Assembly -
- ✓ Mixed green salad - 3 c

- ❖ Mix all dressing ingredients in another container.
- ❖ To make the salad, place the green salad on two plates and cover with the dressing. Drizzle with the dressing and enjoy.

35) Pineapple salad

Preparation time:　　　　Cooking time:　　　　Servings: 1

Ingredients:

- ✓ Seasoning -
- ✓ Chopped cilantro, .5 c.
- ✓ Chopped shallots, .5 c.
- ✓ Lime juice, 2 tablespoons
- ✓ Water, .25 c.
- ✓ Avocado oil, .25 c.
- ✓ Sea salt, 0.5 teaspoons

Directions:

- ❖ Place each seasoning content in your blender and blend until well combined. Adjust seasonings as needed.

Nutrition: Calories

Ingredients:

- ✓ Garlic, 2 cloves
- ✓ Assembly -
- ✓ Dulce flakes
- ✓ Chopped purple cabbage, 1 c.
- ✓ Cubed pineapple, .5 c.
- ✓ Mixed salad, 2 c.

- ❖ To make the salad, place the green salad in a bowl and add the dulse flakes, purple cabbage and pineapple. Pour in the dressing and toss to combine. Enjoy.

36) *Sweet potato salad with Jalapeno sauce*

Preparation time:

Cooking time:

Servings: 2

Ingredients:

- ✓ Sweet potatoes -
- ✓ Sea salt, .25 tsp
- ✓ Paprika, 1 teaspoon
- ✓ Crushed garlic, 2 cloves
- ✓ Avocado oil, 2 tablespoons
- ✓ Sweet potatoes peeled and diced, 3
- ✓ Seasoning -
- ✓ Water, 1 c.

Directions:

- ❖ Start by setting your kitchen appliance to three hundred and fifty degrees. Place some parchment on a sheet of kitchen paper.
- ❖ Dice the sweet potatoes with the salt, paprika, garlic and avocado oil. Make sure the potatoes are well coated.

Ingredients:

- ✓ Sea salt, 0.5 teaspoons
- ✓ Lime juice, 2 tablespoons
- ✓ Jalapeno
- ✓ Cilantro leaves, .25 c.
- ✓ Raw cashews, 1 c.
- ✓ Assembly -
- ✓ Mixed salad, 2 c.

- ❖ Spread the sweet potatoes on the baking sheet and bake for 25 minutes, or until soft.
- ❖ While the potatoes are cooking, add the salt, lime juice, jalapeno, cilantro, cashews and water to a high-speed blender and blend until smooth.
- ❖ To make the salad, divide the green salad into two plates and top with the cooked sweet potatoes. Add the dressing and toss to combine.

Nutrition: Calories

37) *Asparagus salad with lemon sauce*

Preparation time:

Cooking time:

Portions:

Ingredients:

- ✓ Salad -
- ✓ Pepper, .25 tsp
- ✓ Sea salt, 0.5 teaspoons
- ✓ Crushed garlic, 3 cloves
- ✓ Diced onion, .5 c.
- ✓ Diced asparagus stems, 24
- ✓ Avocado oil, 1 teaspoon

Directions:

- ❖ For the asparagus, heat the oil in a massive skillet and put in the pepper, salt, garlic, onion bulb, then the asparagus. Prepare for five to seven minutes, or until the onion has become soft.
- ❖ To make the dressing, add half of the cooked asparagus mixture to a blender along with the pepper, salt, lemon juice, water and cashews.

Nutrition: Calories

Ingredients:

- ✓ Seasoning -
- ✓ Pepper
- ✓ Sea salt, .25 tsp
- ✓ Lemon juice, 2 tablespoons
- ✓ Water, .5 c.
- ✓ Raw cashews, .5 c.
- ✓ Assembly -
- ✓ Mixed salad, 2 c.

- ❖ Blend until smooth and creamy.
- ❖ To make the salad, divide the vegetable mixture between two plates and top with the rest of the cooked asparagus. Top with the dressing and enjoy.

38) Vegetarian lettuce rolls

Preparation time: 20 minutes   **Cooking time**: 10 minutes   **Servings: 4**

Ingredients:

- ✓ For filling:
- ✓ 1 teaspoon of olive oil
- ✓ 2 cups fresh shiitake mushrooms, chopped
- ✓ 2 teaspoons of tamari, divided
- ✓ 1 cup of cooked quinoa
- ✓ 1 teaspoon fresh lime juice
- ✓ 1 teaspoon organic apple cider vinegar
- ✓ ¼ cup shallots, chopped
- ✓ Sea salt and freshly ground black pepper, to taste
- ✓ For the creamy sauce:
- ✓ 5 ounces of silken tofu, pressed, drained and chopped
- ✓ 1 small clove of garlic, minced

Directions:

- ❖ For the filling, in a skillet, heat oil over medium heat and cook mushrooms and 1 teaspoon tamari for about 5-8 minutes, stirring often.
- ❖ Stir in the quinoa, lime juice, vinegar and remaining tamari and cook for about 1 minute, stirring constantly.
- ❖ Add the shallot, salt and black pepper and immediately remove from heat.

Nutrition: Calories

Ingredients:

- ✓ ¼ cup plain almond butter
- ✓ 1 teaspoon fresh lime juice
- ✓ Sea salt and freshly ground black pepper, to taste
- ✓ For wrappers:
- ✓ 8 medium lettuce leaves
- ✓ ¼ cup cucumber, peeled and julienned
- ✓ ¼ cup of carrot, peeled and julienned
- ✓ ¼ cup of cabbage, shredded

- ❖ Set aside to cool.
- ❖ Meanwhile, for the sauce: in a food processor, add all ingredients and pulse until smooth.
- ❖ Arrange the lettuce leaves on serving plates.
- ❖ Place quinoa filling evenly on each leaf and top with cucumbers, carrots and cabbage.
- ❖ Serve alongside the creamy sauce.

39) Oatmeal, tofu and spinach burger

Preparation time: 15 minutes   **Cooking time**: 16 minutes   **Servings: 4**

Ingredients:

- ✓ 1 pound firm tofu, drained, pressed and crumbled
- ✓ ¾ cup rolled oats
- ✓ ¼ cup of flaxseed
- ✓ 2 cups frozen cabbage, thawed, squeezed and shredded
- ✓ 1 medium onion, finely chopped
- ✓ 4 garlic cloves, minced

Directions:

- ❖ In a large bowl, add all ingredients except oil and green salads and mix until well combined.
- ❖ Set aside for about 10 minutes.
- ❖ Cut out desired size patties from the dough.

Nutrition: Calories

Ingredients:

- ✓ 1 teaspoon of ground cumin
- ✓ 1 teaspoon of red pepper flakes, crushed
- ✓ Sea salt and freshly ground black pepper, to taste
- ✓ 2 tablespoons of olive oil
- ✓ 6 cups of fresh salad

- ❖ In a nonstick skillet, heat oil over medium heat and cook patties for 6-8 minutes per side.
- ❖ Serve these patties alongside the green salad.

40) Hamburger with beans, nuts and vegetables

Preparation time: 20 minutes   **Cooking time**: 25 minutes   **Servings: 4**

Ingredients:

- ✓ ½ cup of walnuts
- ✓ 1 carrot, peeled and chopped
- ✓ 1 celery stalk, chopped
- ✓ 4 shallots, chopped
- ✓ 5 cloves of garlic, minced
- ✓ 2¼ cups canned black beans, rinsed and drained

Directions:

- ❖ Preheat oven to 400 degrees F. Line a baking sheet with baking paper.
- ❖ In a food processor, add the walnuts and pulse until finely ground.
- ❖ Add the carrot, celery, shallot and garlic and chop finely.
- ❖ Transfer the vegetable mixture to a large bowl.
- ❖ In the same food processor, add the beans and pulse until chopped.
- ❖ Add 1 1/2 cups sweet potatoes and pulse until a chunky mixture forms.

Nutrition: Calories

Ingredients:

- ✓ 2½ cups sweet potato, peeled and grated
- ✓ ½ teaspoon of red pepper flakes, crushed
- ✓ ¼ teaspoon cayenne pepper
- ✓ Sea salt and freshly ground black pepper, to taste
- ✓ 12 cups of fresh vegetables

- ❖ Transfer the bean mixture to the bowl with the vegetable mixture.
- ❖ Stir in the remaining sweet potato, spices, salt and black pepper and mix until well combined.
- ❖ Make 8 equal-sized patties with the bean mixture.
- ❖ Arrange the meatballs on the prepared baking sheet in a single layer.
- ❖ Bake for about 25 minutes.
- ❖ Divide vegetables among serving plates and top each with 2 meatballs.
- ❖ Serve immediately.

Alkaline Diet Dinner Recipes

41) Potato and broccoli soup

Preparation time: 10 minutes

Cooking time: 25 minutes

Servings: 2 to 1

Ingredients:

- ✓ 1 tablespoon avocado oil
- ✓ ½ cup diced onion
- ✓ 2 garlic cloves, crushed
- ✓ 3 cups of vegetable broth
- ✓ 1 (13.5-ounce / 383-g) can of whole coconut milk

Directions:

- ❖ In a large skillet over medium-high heat, heat the avocado oil. Add the onion and garlic and sauté for 2 to 3 minutes, or until the onions are soft.
- ❖ Add the vegetable broth, coconut milk, potatoes, broccoli, salt and pepper, and continue to cook for 18-20 minutes, or until the potatoes are soft. Remove from heat and cool.

Nutrition: Calories

Ingredients:

- ✓ 2 cups of potatoes peeled and cut into cubes
- ✓ 3 cups chopped broccoli florets
- ✓ 1 teaspoon of sea salt
- ✓ 1½ teaspoons of freshly ground black pepper

- ❖ In a blender, blend the cooled soup until smooth.
- ❖ Adjust seasonings as needed. Pour into 2 large or 4 small bowls and enjoy.

42) Lush bell pepper soup

Preparation time: 5 minutes

Cooking time: 10 minutes

Servings: from 2 to 4

Ingredients:

- ✓ 1 teaspoon of avocado oil
- ✓ ¼ cup diced onions
- ✓ 2 garlic cloves, crushed
- ✓ 2 cups of diced red peppers
- ✓ 2 cups of vegetable broth

Directions:

- ❖ In a skillet over medium-high heat, add avocado oil, onions, garlic, and red peppers, and sauté for 2 to 3 minutes, or until onions are soft; let cool.
- ❖ In a blender, blend together the soffritto, vegetable broth, jalapeño, and salt until well combined and completely liquid; adjust seasonings according to your preference.

Nutrition: Calories

Ingredients:

- ✓ ½ to 1 jalapeño, seeded and diced
- ✓ 1 teaspoon of sea salt
- ✓ ½ cup diced red peppers
- ✓ ½ cup of diced yellow peppers

- ❖ Transfer the soup to a medium bowl and toss with the diced red and yellow peppers.
- ❖ Cover and refrigerate for 20-30 minutes to chill or chill overnight.
- ❖ Pour into 2 large or 4 small bowls and enjoy.

43) Cabbage and yellow onion soup

Preparation time: 10 minutes

Cooking time: 20 minutes

Servings: from 2 to 4

Ingredients:

- ✓ 1 tablespoon avocado oil
- ✓ 2 cups thinly sliced yellow onions (3 medium)
- ✓ 1 teaspoon of unrefined whole cane sugar, such as Sucanat
- ✓ 1 cup of vegetable broth
- ✓ 2 cups of water

Directions:

- ❖ In a medium saucepan over medium-high heat, heat the avocado oil. Add the onions and sauté for 3-5 minutes, or until the onions begin to get soft.
- ❖ Add the sugar and continue to sauté, stirring constantly, for 8-10 minutes, or until the onions are slightly caramelized.

Nutrition: Calories

Ingredients:

- ✓ 2 tablespoons of coconut amino acids
- ✓ 2 garlic cloves, crushed
- ✓ ½ teaspoon of dried thyme
- ✓ ½ teaspoon of sea salt
- ✓ 3 cabbage stalks, shredded and cut into ribbons (about 2 cups)
- ❖ Add the vegetable broth, water, coconut amino acid, garlic, thyme, and salt. Reduce heat to medium-low and simmer for 5-7 minutes. Adjust seasonings as needed.
- ❖ Add the cabbage and leave on the heat just long enough to wilt it.
- ❖ Remove from heat, pour into 2 large or 4 small bowls and serve.

44) Wild rice, mushroom and leek soup

Preparation time: 10 minutes   **Cooking time:** 55 minutes   **Servings: 1 to 2**

Ingredients:

- ✓ ⅓ cup of wild rice
- ✓ 1 cup sliced cremini mushrooms
- ✓ ½ cup sliced leeks, white part only
- ✓ 3 cups of water

Directions:

- ❖ Prepare wild rice according to package instructions.
- ❖ In a medium saucepan over high heat, bring sliced mushrooms, leeks and water to a boil. Boil for 8-10 minutes, or until mushrooms are soft.

Nutrition: Calories

Ingredients:

- ✓ 2 tablespoons of organic white miso
- ✓ ¼ to ½ teaspoon freshly ground black pepper
- ✓ Sliced shallots, for garnish

- ❖ Add the cooked wild rice, miso and black pepper. Using the back side of a spoon, mash the miso on the side of the pot to break it up, then stir it in.
- ❖ Remove from heat. Pour into 1 large or 2 small bowls, garnish with chopped scallions and enjoy.

45) Pear and ginger soup

Preparation time: 10 minutes   **Cooking time:** 15 minutes   **Servings: 1 to 2**

Ingredients:

- ✓ 2 teaspoons of avocado oil
- ✓ ½ cup diced onions
- ✓ 2 garlic cloves, crushed
- ✓ 1 cup of vegetable broth
- ✓ 2 cups of water
- ✓ ¼ cup coconut milk (canned)

Directions:

- ❖ In a large skillet over medium-high heat, heat the avocado oil. Add the onion and garlic and sauté for 2 to 3 minutes, or until the onions are soft.
- ❖ Add the vegetable broth, water, coconut milk, pears, ginger and salt, and cook over medium-high heat for 8-10 minutes, or until the pears are soft. Remove from heat and cool.

Nutrition: Calories

Ingredients:

- ✓ 2 pears peeled and cut into cubes
- ✓ 1 inch fresh ginger root, chopped
- ✓ ¼ teaspoon of sea salt
- ✓ Sliced radishes, for garnish (optional)
- ✓ Chopped shallots, for garnish (optional)

- ❖ Transfer the soup to a blender and blend until well combined. Adjust seasonings as needed.
- ❖ Pour immediately into 1 large bowl or 2 small bowls, garnish with the radishes and scallions (if using), and enjoy, or return the soup to the stove to warm slightly over low heat before serving.

46) Asparagus and artichoke soup

Preparation time: 5 minutes   **Cooking time:** 20 minutes   **Servings: 4 cups**

Ingredients:

- ✓ ½ cup diced onion
- ✓ 1 tablespoon avocado oil
- ✓ 2 garlic cloves, crushed
- ✓ 1 cup of diced potatoes
- ✓ 8 asparagus stalks, cut into small pieces

Directions:

- ❖ In a medium skillet, sauté onion, avocado oil and garlic over medium-high heat for 2 to 3 minutes, or until onion is soft.
- ❖ Transfer the sauté to a medium-sized saucepan and add the potatoes, asparagus, vegetable broth, salt and pepper; cook over medium-high heat for 18 to 20 minutes, or until the potatoes are soft. Add more vegetable broth, if necessary, to keep the liquid level between ½ and 1 inch above the contents of the saucepan. Remove from heat and allow to cool.

Nutrition: Calories

Ingredients:

- ✓ 2 cups of vegetable broth
- ✓ ½ to ¾ teaspoon sea salt
- ✓ ½ teaspoon of ground black pepper
- ✓ 2 cups of almond milk
- ✓ 1 can of artichoke hearts, cut in half and with stem
- ❖ In a blender, blend the cooled soup mixture, almond milk and artichokes until everything is well combined and the soup is smooth. Adjust the seasonings to your liking and add more almond milk or vegetable broth to thin it out, if you prefer.
- ❖ Return the soup to the casserole dish and heat slightly over low heat before serving.

47) Carrot and celery soup

Preparation time: 15 minutes   **Cooking time:** 1 hour and 10 minutes   **Servings: 4 people**

Ingredients:

- ✓ Kitchen spray
- ✓ 1 large onion, coarsely chopped
- ✓ 2 large carrots, peeled and roughly chopped
- ✓ 2 large celery stalks (with leaves), coarsely chopped
- ✓ 1 parsnip, peeled and coarsely chopped

Ingredients:

- ✓ 5 cloves of garlic, crushed
- ✓ 1 leek, well cleaned and coarsely chopped
- ✓ 9 cups of water
- ✓ 2 bay leaves
- ✓ 2 teaspoons of sea salt
- ❖ Add the water, bay leaf and salt. Simmer for 1 hour.
- ❖ Remove from heat and cool slightly. Drain the vegetables, leaving only the broth.
- ❖ To serve, add back some of the vegetables if you like and heat the soup to your desired temperature.

Directions:

- ❖ Spray the bottom of a large pot with cooking spray. Place the pot over medium-low heat, add the onion and sauté for about 5 minutes, stirring constantly.
- ❖ Add the carrots, celery, parsnips, garlic and leek to the pot. Sauté for an additional 3 minutes.

Nutrition: Calories

48) Creamy clam chowder with mushrooms

Preparation time: 15 minutes   **Cooking time:** 30 minutes   **Servings: 4**

Ingredients:

-    For the mushroom clams:
- ✓ ½ cup coarsely chopped shiitake mushrooms
- ✓ 1 teaspoon of coconut oil
- ✓ ¼ cup of water
- ✓ ½ teaspoon celery seeds
-    For the soup base:
- ✓ ½ medium onion, chopped
- ✓ 3 medium carrots, peeled and chopped
- ✓ 2 stalks of celery, finely chopped

Ingredients:

- ✓ 1 teaspoon of dried thyme
- ✓ 3 cups of vegetable broth
- ✓ 1 sheet of nori, finely crumbled
-    For the cream base:
- ✓ 1 cup lightly steamed cauliflower
- ✓ ¾ cup unsweetened almond milk
- ✓ ¼ teaspoon of sea salt

Directions:

- ❖ To make clams with mushrooms
- ❖ In a large pot over medium-high heat, add mushrooms and coconut oil. Sauté for 3 minutes. Add the water and celery seeds, stirring until the water is absorbed.
- ❖ Remove from heat and transfer mushrooms to a plate.
- ❖ To make the soup base
- ❖ In the same pot, over medium heat, sauté the onion, carrots, celery and thyme for about 5 minutes, or until the onion is softened. Add a little broth, if needed.

- ❖ Then, add the remaining broth and nori and bring to a boil.
- ❖ To make the cream base
- ❖ In a blender or food processor, add the cauliflower, almond milk and salt. Blend to combine. If the mixture is too thick, add a little soup base to thin it out. Blend until the mixture is smooth.
- ❖ To assemble the fish soup
- ❖ Add the mushroom mix and cream base to the soup base. Stir well to combine.
- ❖ Reheat for 5 minutes, or until hot, and serve.

Nutrition: Calories

49) Soup of bok choy, broccolini and brown rice

Preparation time: 5 minutes   **Cooking time:** 10 minutes   **Servings: 2**

Ingredients:

- ✓ 3 cups of vegetable broth
- ✓ 1 cup of chopped bok choy

Ingredients:

- ✓ 1 bunch of broccolini, coarsely chopped
- ✓ ½ cup cooked brown rice

Directions:

- ❖ In a medium saucepan over medium heat, place the broth, bok choy, broccolini and brown rice. Bring to a boil and cook for 10 minutes, or until vegetables are cooked through and tender. Serve.

Nutrition: Calories

50) Apple and sweet pumpkin soup

Preparation time: 5 minutes   **Cooking time:** 25 minutes   **Servings:** 2 people

Ingredients:

- ✓ 1 medium apple, core and slices
- ✓ ½ cup chopped fennel
- ✓ 1½ cups of water, divided
- ✓ 1 cup unsweetened canned pumpkin puree
- ✓ ¾ cup low-sodium vegetable broth
- ✓ 4 small dates, pitted
- ✓ 2 teaspoons of fresh grated ginger or 2 cubes of frozen ginger

Directions:

- ❖ In a saucepan, combine the apples, fennel and ½ cup water. Cover and simmer for about 25 minutes, until the apples and fennel are softened.
- ❖ In a food processor, combine the apple and fennel mixture, pumpkin, remaining 1 cup water, broth, dates, ginger, cinnamon, curry powder, thyme, salt and cumin. Process until reduced to a puree.

Nutrition: Calories

Ingredients:

- ✓ ¼ teaspoon ground cinnamon
- ✓ ¼ teaspoon of curry powder
- ✓ ⅛ teaspoon of dried thyme
- ✓ ⅛ teaspoon sea salt
- ✓ ⅛ teaspoon of ground cumin
- ✓ 4 teaspoons of raisins, for garnish
- ✓ 2 teaspoons fennel seeds, toasted, for garnish
- ❖ Pour soup into two bowls and top each with 2 teaspoons raisins and 1 teaspoon toasted fennel seeds.
- ❖ Serve immediately or let cool and serve at room temperature.

51) Tomato and carrot soup with lemon

Preparation time: 5 minutes   **Cooking time:** 35 minutes   **Servings:** 2

Ingredients:

- ✓ 1(15-ounce / 425-g) can no sodium added diced tomatoes, drained
- ✓ ¾ cup chopped carrots
- ✓ 1 tablespoon avocado oil
- ✓ ¼ teaspoon of sea salt

Directions:

- ❖ Preheat the oven to 400ºF (205ºC).
- ❖ In a glass baking dish, combine the tomatoes, carrots, oil and salt and mix well.

Nutrition: Calories

Ingredients:

- ✓ 1 cup of water
- ✓ ½ cup low-sodium vegetable broth
- ✓ 2 tablespoons fresh coriander chopped
- ✓ 1 tablespoon freshly squeezed lemon juice

- ❖ Cook tomato and carrot mixture for 35 minutes, or until caramelized, then carefully transfer to a food processor.
- ❖ Add the water and broth and blend until smooth.
- ❖ Garnish with the cilantro and add lemon juice to taste.

52) Zucchini and avocado soup with basil

Preparation time: 5 minutes   **Cooking time:** 0 minutes   **Servings:** 2 people

Ingredients:

- ✓ 2 large zucchini, chopped
- ✓ 1 medium avocado
- ✓ 1 medium bell pepper
- ✓ ½ cup low-sodium vegetable broth
- ✓ ½ cup of water
- ✓ ¼ cup chopped fennel

Directions:

- ❖ In a high-speed blender or food processor, combine the zucchini, avocado, bell bell pepper, broth, water, fennel, basil, rosemary, garlic and salt and blend until pureed.

Nutrition: Calories

Ingredients:

- ✓ 6 fresh basil leaves, plus 2 small leaves for garnish
- ✓ 2 teaspoons fresh rosemary chopped
- ✓ 1 garlic clove, peeled, or 1 frozen garlic cube
- ✓ ¼ teaspoon sea salt
- ✓ 1½ teaspoons hulled pumpkin seeds, toasted, for garnish

- ❖ Pour the soup into the bowls. Garnish each with a small basil leaf and the pumpkin seeds and serve.

53) Zucchini, spinach and quinoa soup

Preparation time: 5 minutes   **Cooking time**: 25 minutes   **Servings**: 4 people

Ingredients:

- ✓ 2 tablespoons of avocado oil
- ✓ ¼ teaspoon of dried oregano
- ✓ ¼ teaspoon of dried thyme
- ✓ ⅛ teaspoon sea salt
- ✓ 1 large onion, chopped
- ✓ 2 large zucchini, peeled and cut into pieces

Directions:

- ❖ In a soup pot, heat the oil over medium heat for 1 minute, then add the oregano, thyme and salt and cook for 30 seconds.
- ❖ Add onion, cover and cook for 7-8 minutes, stirring regularly, until softened.
- ❖ Add the zucchini. Cook for an additional 12 minutes, or until zucchini is soft.

Nutrition: Calories

Ingredients:

- ✓ 1 cup low-sodium vegetable broth
- ✓ 1 cup of water
- ✓ 1 cup baby spinach
- ✓ 6 large fresh basil leaves
- ✓ ⅓ cup of cooked quinoa (optional)
- ✓ Juice of 1 lemon
- ❖ Add the broth and water and cook for another 3 minutes, until heated through.
- ❖ Add the spinach and basil and cook until just wilted.
- ❖ Transfer the mixture to a food processor and process until pureed.
- ❖ Add quinoa (if using). Season with lemon juice and serve.

54) Easy Cilantro Lime Quinoa.

Preparation time: 5 minutes   **Cooking time**: 15 minutes   **Servings**: 6

Ingredients:

- ✓ 1 cup quinoa, rinsed and draned.
- ✓ ½ cup fresh cilantro, chopped
- ✓ 1 lime zest, grated

Directions:

- ❖ Add quinoa and water to the instant pot and stir well.
- ❖ Seal with a lid and select manual mode and set the timer for 5 minutes.

Nutrition: Calories

Ingredients:

- ✓ 2 tbsp. fresh lime juice
- ✓ 1 ¼ cup of distilled water feed Sea sa sa

- ❖ Once finished, allow pressure naturally release that open thed.
- ❖ Stir in water, let stand and let rest.
- ❖ Season with salt and serve.

55) Spinach Quinoa

Preparation time: 10 minutes   **Cooking time**: 25 minutes   **Servings**: 4

Ingredients:

- ✓ 1 cup quinoa
- ✓ 2 cups fresh spinach, chopped
- ✓ 1 ½ cups filtered alkaline water
- ✓ 1 sweet potato, peeled and cut into pieces
- ✓ 1 tsp. coriander powder
- ✓ 1 teaspoon of turmandine
- ✓ 1 teaspoon of cumin seds

Directions:

- ❖ Add oil il instant pot and set the sauté mode.
- ❖ Add onion in olive oil and saute for 2 minutes otil onion is softened.
- ❖ Add garlic, ginger, spices and quinoa and coook for 3-4 minutes.
- ❖ Add spinach, sweet potatoes, and water and stir well.

Nutrition: Calories

Ingredients:

- ✓ 1 tsp. fresh ginger, chopped
- ✓ 2 garlic cloves, chopped
- ✓ 1 onion cut in half
- ✓ 2 tbsp olive oil
- ✓ 1 fresh lime juice
- ✓ Pepper Salt

- ❖ Cook on high pressure for 2 minutes.
- ❖ When it's finished, release the pressure naturally and then open the container. Add the lime juice and mix well.
- ❖ Serve and enjoy.

56) Healthy broccoli soup Asparagus

Preparation time: 15 minutes.   **Cooking time:** 28 minutes.   **Servings:** 6

Ingredients:

- ✓ 2 cups broccoli florets, chopped
- ✓ 15 asparagus spears, es cut and chopped
- ✓ 1 tsp. dried oregano
- ✓ 1 tbsp. fresh thyme leaves
- ✓ ½ cup unsweetened almond milk

Directions:

- ❖ Add the oil to the bowl and stir the bowl.
- ❖ Add onion to olive oil and sauté until onion is softened.
- ❖ Add the garlic and let stand for 30 minutes.
- ❖ Add all the vegetables and salt and dry well.

Nutrition: Calories

Ingredients:

- ✓ 3 ½ cups filtered alkaline water
- ✓ 2 cups cauliflower florets, chopped
- ✓ 2 tsp. garlic, chopped 1 cup onion, chopped
- ✓ 2 tbsp. olive oil
- ✓ Salt Pepper
- ❖ Seal pot with lid and coook on manual mode for 3 minutes.
- ❖ Once finished, you can rinse to minimize pressure and then close the container.
- ❖ Puree the soup with an immersion blender until smooth. Add the almond milk, herbs, pepper and salt.
- ❖ Serve and enjoy.

57) Creamy Asparagus Soup

Preparation time: 10 minutes   **Cooking time:** 40 minutes   **Servings:** 6

Ingredients:

- ✓ 2 lbs. fresh asparagus cut off woody stems
- ✓ ¼ tablespoon of lemon zest
- ✓ 2 tbsp. lime juice
- ✓ 14 oz. coconut milk
- ✓ 1 tsp. tied thyme.
- ✓ ½ tsp. oregano
- ✓ ½ tsp. sage

Directions:

- ❖ Preheat the oven to 400°F/ 200°C.
- ❖ The paper tray with the scraps and leftovers.
- ❖ Arrange the asparagus spears on a baking sheet. Add 2 tablespoons of walnut oil and add salt, seasonings, garlic and sugar.
- ❖ Kiss it with a dose of 20-25 mnutes.
- ❖ Add the remaining oil in the instant pot and set the pot on sauté mode.
- ❖ Add the garlic and milk to the pot and saute for 2-3 minutes.

Nutrition: Calories

Ingredients:

- ✓ 1 ½ cups alkaline water filtered.
- ✓ 1 Head of a hunting dog coming out of the floor.
- ✓ 1 tablespoon. garlic, minced
- ✓ 1 leek, sliced
- ✓ 3 tbsp. coconut oil
- ✓ Pinch of Himalayan salt.

- ❖ Add the cauliflower florets and water to the bowl and mix well.
- ❖ Insert pot with a rod and select steam and let stand for 4 minutes.
- ❖ When you finished, release the pressure using the quick-release method.
- ❖ Add roasted asparagus, lime zest, lime juice, and coco milk and stir well.
- ❖ Puree the soup with an immersion blender until pureed.
- ❖ Serve and have fun

58) Spicy Eggplant

Preparation time: 15 minutes   **Cooking time:** 5 minutes   **Servings:** 4

Ingredients:

- ✓ 1 eggplant, cut into 1inch cubes
- ✓ ½ cup filtered alkaline water
- ✓ 1 life, in book form.
- ✓ ½ tsp. Italian seasoning
- ✓ 1 tsp. paprika

Directions:

- ❖ Add the extract and salt to the instant flour.
- ❖ Cook on manual high pressure for 5 minutes.
- ❖ When done, rinse with peanut butter and then milk. Wet eggplant well.

Nutrition: Calories

Ingredients:

- ✓ ½ tsp. red pepper
- ✓ 1 tsp. garlic powder
- ✓ 2 tbsp. olive oil extra virgin
- ✓ ¼ teaspoon of sea salt

- ❖ Add oil to the Instant Pot and set pot on sauté mode.
- ❖ Return the ingredient to the pot with the food processor, garlic, paprika, red, garlic and salt and stir until included.
- ❖ Coook on sauté mode for 5 minutes. Stir from time to time.
- ❖ Serve enjoy.

59) Brussels Sprouts and carrots

Preparation time: 10 minutes   **Cooking time**: 5 minutes   **Servings**: 6

Ingredients:

- ✓ 1 1/2 pounds of Brussels sprouts, trimmed and cut alf
- ✓ 4 Carrots peel and cut slices are shaped into a knife.
- ✓ 1 tsp. olive oil
- ✓ ½ cup alkaline filtered water
- ✓ 1 tbsp. dried parsley

Directions:

- ❖ Add all ingredients inside the instant pot and mix well.
- ❖ Cook the pot with the lid on and cook on high heat for 2 minutes.

Nutrition: Calories

Ingredients:

- ✓ ¼ tsp. garlic, chopped
- ✓ ¼ tsp. pepper
- ✓ ¼ tsp. sea salt

- ❖ When finished, rinse with the quick release button and then the lid.
- ❖ Stir well all and serve.

60) Cajun Zucchini seasoned

Preparation time: 8 minutes.   **Cooking time**: 2 minutes.   **Servings**: 2

Ingredients:

- ✓ 4 zucchinis, sliced
- ✓ 1 tsp. garlic powder
- ✓ 1 tsp. paprika

Directions:

- ❖ Add all ingredients to the pot and mix well.
- ❖ Close the pot with the lid and cook on low pressure for 1 minute.
- ❖ Nutrition: Calories 130 Fat: 7.9 Carbohydrates: 14.7 g. Sugar: 7.2 g. Protein: 5.3 g. Cholesterol: 0 mg.

Ingredients:

- ✓ 2 tbsp. Cajun seasoning
- ✓ ½ cup melted milk water
- ✓ 1 tablespoon of olive oil

- ❖ Once finished, release the pressure using the quick-release method then opene the lid.
- ❖ Mix well and serve.

61) Cracker Healthy

Preparation time: **Cooking time:** 30 minutes **Servings:** 50 Crackers

Ingredients:
- ✓ 1/2 cup of rye flour
- ✓ 1 cup of flour Spelt
- ✓ 2 teaspoons of Sesame Seed
- ✓ 1 teaspoon of Agave Syrup

Directions:
- ❖ Preheat our oven to 350 degrees Fahrenheit.
- ❖ Add all ingredients to a glass container and mix everything together.
- ❖ Make a ball of dough. If the dough is too thick, add more flour.
- ❖ Prepare a place to spread the dough and cover it with a piece of parchment paper.
- ❖ Degrease the container well with Grape Seed Oil and put the dart in it.
- ❖ RICE the slurry with a rolling pin, adding more flour so it doesn't fall apart.

Ingredients:
- ✓ 1 teaspoon of Pure Sea Salt
- ✓ 2 tablespoons of Grape Seed Oil
- ✓ 3/4 cup of Spring Water

- ❖ When your dough is ready, take a pastry cutter and insert it into the container. If you don't have a pastry cutter, you can use a cookie cutter.
- ❖ Arrange the squares on a kitchen basket and place them in the corner of a ech square using a fork of a skewer.
- ❖ Brush the plate with a little grain oil and sprinkle with a little pure sea salt, if needed.
- ❖ Bake for 12-15 minutes or until crackers are golden brown.
- ❖ Everything that was done was done with the help of another person.
- ❖ Serve and enjoy your Healthy Crackers!

62) Tortillas

Preparation time:. **Cooking Time:** 20 Minutes **Servings:** 8

Ingredients:
- ✓ 2 cups of flour Spelt
- ✓ 1 teaspoon of Pure Sea Salt

Directions:
- ❖ In a food processor* blend the spelt flour with the pure salt. Blend for about 15 minutes.
- ❖ Blend, slowly add Grape seed oil until well distributed.
- ❖ Slowly add the soy water, stirring until a color forms.
- ❖ Prepare a piece of wallpaper and pour some parchment paper on it. Dust with a little flour.

Ingredients:
- ✓ 1/2 cup of spring Water

- ❖ Process the nut for about 1 to 2 minutes until it reaches the right consistency.
- ❖ Pour dough into 8-inch pieces.
- ❖ Roll the sandwich into a very thin shape.
- ❖ Prepare a lunch box, cook one tortilla at a time in the microwave for about 30-60 minutes.
- ❖ Serve and enjoy your Tortillas!

63) Walnut cheesecake Mango

Preparation time: **Cooking time:** 4 hours and 30 minutes **Servings:** 8

Ingredients:
- ✓ 2 cups of Brazil Nuts
- ✓ 5 to 6 Dates
- ✓ 1 tablespoon of Sea Moss Gel (check information)
- ✓ 1/4 cup o of agave syrup
- ✓ 1/4 teaspoon salt Pure Sea
- ✓ 2 tablespoons of Lime Juice
- ✓ 1 1/2 cups of Homemade Walnut Milk *

Directions:
- ❖ Place all crust ingredients in a processor and blend for 30 seconds.
- ❖ Prepare a baking sheet with a sheet of parchment and roll out the loose dough with butter.
- ❖ Place the Mango sliced across the crust and freeze for 10 minutes.
- ❖ Place all the glass pieces in a bowl until ready.

Ingredients:
- **Crust:**
- ✓ 1 1/2 cups of quartered Dates 1/4 cup of Agave Syrup
- ✓ 1 1/2 cups of Coconut Flakes
- ✓ 1/4 teaspoon of Pure Sea Salt
- ✓ **Toppings:**
- ✓ Mango of Sliced
- ✓ Sliced strawberries
- ❖ Place the filling on top of the butter, wrap it with aluminum foil or a food container and let it rest for 3 to 4 hours in the refrigerator.
- ❖ Take out dalla baking form and garnish with toppings.
- ❖ Serve and enjoy our Mango Nut Cheesecake!

64) Blackberry Jam

Preparation time: **Cooking time:** 4 hours and 30 minutes   **Servings:** 1 cup

Ingredients:

- ✓ 3/4 cup of Blackberries
- ✓ 1 tablespoon lime juice Key

Directions:

- ❖ Place blackberries in a medium saucepan and cook over low heat.
- ❖ Stir in blackberries until liquid is gone.
- ❖ Once you've picked the berries, use your blender to chop up the larger pieces. If you don't have a blender, put the mixture in an immersion blender, blend it well, and then return it to the oven.

Ingredients:

- ✓ 3 tablespoons of Agave Syrup
- ✓ ¼ cup of Sea Moss Gel + extra 2 tablespoons (check information)

- ❖ Add Sea Moss Gel, Key Lime Juice and Agave Syrup to the mixture. Cook over low heat and stir well until dry.
- ❖ Remove from heat and let sit for 10 minutes.
- ❖ Serve with pieces on flat bread.
- ❖ Enjoy your jam!

65) Blackberry Bars

Preparation time: **Cooking time:** 1 hour 20 Minutes   **Servings:** 4

Ingredients:

- ✓ 3 Burro Banas or 4 Baby Banas
- ✓ 1 cup of Spelt Flour
- ✓ 2 cups of Quinoa Flakes
- ✓ 1/4 cup of Agave Syrup

Directions:

- ❖ Set the oven to 350 degrees Fahrenheit.
- ❖ Mash the bananas with a fork in a large bowl.
- ❖ Combine Agave Syrup and Grape Seed Oil to the puree and mix well.
- ❖ Add the Spelt flour and Quinoa flakes. Knead the dough until it becomes sticky to your finger.
- ❖ Prepare a 9x9-inch basket with a parchment lid.
- ❖ Take 2/3 of the dough and spread it with your fingers on the baking sheet parchment pan.

.

Ingredients:

- ✓ 1/4 teaspoon of Pure Sea Salt
- ✓ 1/2 cup of Grape Seed Oil
- ✓ 1 cup of prepared Blackberry Jam

- ❖ Spread Blackberry Jam over the dough.
- ❖ Crumble the rice and place it on the plate.
- ❖ Bake for 20 minutes.
- ❖ Remove from oven and let cool for 10-15 minutes.
- ❖ Cut into small pieces.
- ❖ Try and enjoy our Blackberry Bars!

66) Squash Pie.

Preparation time: **Cooking time:** 2 hours 30 Minutes   **Servings:** 6-8

Ingredients:

- ✓ 2 Butternut Squashes
- ✓ 1 1/4 cups of spelt flour
- ✓ 1/4 cup of dry sugar
- ✓ 1/4 cup of Agave Syrup
- ✓ 1 teaspoon of Allspice.

Directions:

- ❖ Rinse and peel butternut pumpkins.
- ❖ Cut them in half and use a spoon to de-sed.
- ❖ Cut the meat into one piece and place in a glass container.
- ❖ Cover the squash in Spring Water and boiltare for 20-25 minutes until coooked.
- ❖ Turn off the oven and mash the cooked squash.
- ❖ Add the date sugar, agave syrup, 1/8 pure sea salt, and homemade milk and mix everything together.
- ❖ Crust:
- ❖ Preheat the oven to 350 degrees Fahrenheit.
- ❖ In a bowl, add the spelt flour, 1/2 teaspoon of Pure Sea Salt, Spring Water, and Grape Sed Oil and mix.

Ingredients:

- ✓ 1 teaspoon of Pure Sea Salt
- ✓ 1/4 cup soy water
- ✓ 1/3 cup of fat seed oil
- ✓ 1/4 cup hemp seed milk Homemade *

- ❖ Reduce the rice into a loaf of bread. Add more water or flour if needed. Let stand for 5 minutes.
- ❖ Spread out Spelt Flour on a piece of parchment paper.
- ❖ Roll out on rolling pin, adding more flour to prevent sticking.
- ❖ Place the dough in a cake pan and bake for 10 minutes.
- ❖ Remove the butter from the oven, add the filling and bake for another 40 minutes.
- ❖ Remove the cake and let it rest for 30 minutes until cool.
- ❖ Serve enjoy your Squash Pie!

67) Walnut Milk homemade

Preparation time:

Cooking time: minimum 8 hours

Servings: 4 cups

Ingredients:
- ✓ 1 cup fresh walnuts
- ✓ 1/8 teaspoon of Pure Sea Salt

Directions:
- ❖ Place the new Walnuts in a bag and fill it with three tablespoons of water.
- ❖ Take the Walnuts for an hour and a half.
- ❖ Drain and rinse nuts with warm water.

Ingredients:
- ✓ 3 cups of spring water + extra for soaking

- ❖ Add the soaked walnuts, puree and three times the spring water to a blender.
- ❖ Mix well till smooth.
- ❖ Extend it if you need to.
- ❖ Enjoy your homemade nut milk!

68) Aquafaba

Preparation time:

Cooking time: 2 Hours 30 minutes

Servings: 2-4 cups

Ingredients:
- ✓ 1 bag of Garbanzo beans
- ✓ 1 teaspoon of Pure Sea Salt

Directions:
- ❖ Place the chickpeas in a large pot, add the soy water and pure sea salt. Bring to a boil.
- ❖ Remove from heat and allow to soak 30 to 40 minutes.
- ❖ Strain the Garbanzo Beans and add 6 cups of water.
- ❖ Boil for 1 hour and 30 minutes on medium hat.

Ingredients:
- ✓ 6 cups of Spring Water + extra for soaking

- ❖ Filter the Garbanzo beans. This filtered water is Aquafaba.
- ❖ Pour the Aquafaba into a glass jar with a lid and place in the refrigerator.
- ❖ After cooling, the Aquafaba becomes thicker. If it is too thick, boil for 10-20 mnutes.

69) Milk Homemade Hempsed

Preparation time:

Cooking time: 2 hours

Servings: 2 cups

Ingredients:
- ✓ 2 tablespoons of Hemp Seeds
- ✓ 2 tablespoons of Agave Syrup

Directions:
- ❖ Place all ingredients, except fruit, in blender.
- ❖ Blend them for two minutes.
- ❖ Add fruits and resin for 30-50 minutes.

Nutrition: Calories

Helpful Hints:

Ingredients:
- ✓ 1/8 teaspoon pure salt
- ✓ 2 cups of Spring Water Fruits (optional)*.

- ❖ Store milk in the refrigerator until aged.
- ❖ Enjoy your Homemade Hempsed Milk!

70) Oil spicy infusion

Preparation time:

Cooking time: 24 Hours

Servings: 1 cup

Ingredients:

- ✓ *1 tablespoon of crushed Cayenne Pepper*

Directions:
- ❖ Fill a glass with a lid or bottle with grape oil.
- ❖ Add crushed Cayenne Pepper to the jar/bottle.

Ingredients:
- ✓ 3/4 cup of Grape Seed Oil

- ❖ Close and allow to cool for at least 24 hours.
- ❖ Add it to a dinner party and enjoy our Spicy Infuse oil!

71) Italian infused oil

Preparation time: Cooking time: 24 hours   Servings: 1 cup

Ingredients:

- ✓ 1 teaspoon of Oregano.
- ✓ 1 teaspoon of Basil

Directions:

- ❖ Fill a glass jar with a lid or container with grape oil.
- ❖ Mix the seasonings and add them to the rice and lettuce.

Nutrition: Calories

Helpful Hints:

Ingredients:

- ✓ 1 pinch of salt Pure Sea
- ✓ 3/4 cup of Grape seed oil

- ❖ Shake and let the oil steep for at least 24 hours.
- ❖ Add it to a dish and enjoy your Infused Oil Italian!

72) Garlic Infused Oil

Preparation time: Cooking time: 24 hours   Servings: 1 cup

Ingredients:

- ✓ 1/2 teaspoon of Dill
- ✓ 1/2 teaspoon of Ginger Powder
- ✓ 1 tablespoon of Onion Powder.

Directions:

- ❖ Fill a glass jar or squeeze bottle with grapeseed oil.
- ❖ Add the seasonings to the jar/bottle.

Ingredients:

- ✓ 1/2 teaspoon of Pure Sea Salt
- ✓ 3/4 cup of fat seed oil

- ❖ Close and let oil infuse for at least 24 hours.
- ❖ Add it to a dish and add your "Garlic". Infused Oil!

73) Papaya Seeds Mango Dressing

Preparation time: Cooking time: 10 minutes   Servings: 1/2 Cup

Ingredients:

- ✓ 1 cup of chopped Mango
- ✓ 1 teaspoon of Papaya Seeds Ground
- ✓ 1 teaspoon of Basil
- ✓ 1 teaspoon of Onion Powder

Directions:

- ❖ Prepare and place all ingredients into the mixture.
- ❖ Blend for one minute until smoth.

Nutrition: Calories

Helpful Hints:

Ingredients:

- ✓ 1 teaspoon of Agave Syrup
- ✓ 2 tablespoons of lemon juice
- ✓ 1/4 cup of grape oil
- ✓ 1/4 teaspoon salt Pure Sea
- ❖ Add it to a dish and enjoy our Papaya Seed Mango Dress5ng!

74) Blueberry Smoothie

Preparation time: 10 minutes   Cooking time: Servings: 2

Ingredients:

- ✓ 2 cups of frozen blueberries
- ✓ 1 small banana

Directions:

- ❖ Place all ingredients in a high speed blender and pulse until creamy.

Ingredients:

- ✓ 1½ cups unsweetened almond milk
- ✓ ¼ cup ice cubes
- ❖ Pour the smoothie into two glasses and serve immediately.

75) _Raspberry and tofu smoothie_

Preparation time: 10 minutes   Cooking time: Servings: 2

Ingredients:

- ✓ 1½ cups of fresh raspberries
- ✓ 6 ounces of firm silken tofu, pressed and drained
- ✓ 4-5 drops of liquid stevia

Directions:

- ❖ Place all ingredients in a high speed blender and pulse until creamy.

Nutrition: Calories

Helpful Hints:

Ingredients:

- ✓ 1 cup of coconut cream
- ✓ ¼ cup ice, crushed

- ❖ Pour the smoothie into two glasses and serve immediately.

76) _Beet and Strawberry Smoothie_

Preparation time: 10 minutes   Cooking time: Servings: 2

Ingredients:

- ✓ 2 cups frozen strawberries, pitted and chopped
- ✓ ⅔ cup roasted and frozen beet, chopped
- ✓ 1 teaspoon fresh ginger, peeled and grated

Directions:

- ❖ Place all ingredients in a high speed blender and pulse until creamy.

Nutrition: Calories

Helpful Hints:

Ingredients:

- ✓ 1 teaspoon fresh turmeric, peeled and grated
- ✓ ½ cup of fresh orange juice
- ✓ 1 cup unsweetened almond milk

- ❖ Pour the smoothie into two glasses and serve immediately.

77) _Kiwi Smoothie_

Preparation time: 10 minutes   Cooking time: Servings: 2

Ingredients:

- ✓ 4 kiwis
- ✓ 2 small bananas, peeled
- ✓ 1½ cups unsweetened almond milk

Directions:

- ❖ Place all ingredients in a high speed blender and pulse until creamy.

Nutrition: Calories

Helpful Hints:

Ingredients:

- ✓ 1-2 drops of liquid stevia
- ✓ ¼ cup ice cubes

- ❖ Pour the smoothie into two glasses and serve immediately.

78) _Pineapple and Carrot Smoothie_

Preparation time: 10 minutes   Cooking time: Servings: 2

Ingredients:

- ✓ 1 cup frozen pineapple
- ✓ 1 large ripe banana, peeled and sliced
- ✓ ½ tablespoon fresh ginger, peeled and chopped
- ✓ ¼ teaspoon ground turmeric

Directions:

- ❖ Place all ingredients in a high speed blender and pulse until creamy.

Nutrition: Calories

Helpful Hints:

Ingredients:

- ✓ 1 cup unsweetened almond milk
- ✓ ½ cup fresh carrot juice
- ✓ 1 tablespoon fresh lemon juice

- ❖ Pour the smoothie into two glasses and serve immediately.

79) Oatmeal and orange smoothie

Preparation time: 10 minutes   **Cooking time**:   **Servings**: 4

Ingredients:

- ✓ ⅔ cup of rolled oats
- ✓ 2 oranges, peeled, seeds removed and cut into sections
- ✓ 2 large bananas, peeled and sliced

Directions:

- ❖ Place all ingredients in a high speed blender and pulse until creamy.

Nutrition: Calories

Helpful Hints:

Ingredients:

- ✓ 2 cups of unsweetened almond milk
- ✓ 1 cup ice cubes, crushed

- ❖ Pour the smoothie into four glasses and serve immediately.

80) Pumpkin Smoothie

Preparation time: 10 minutes   **Cooking time**:   **Servings**: 2

Ingredients:

- ✓ 1 cup homemade pumpkin puree
- ✓ 1 medium banana, peeled and sliced
- ✓ 1 tablespoon maple syrup
- ✓ 1 teaspoon ground flax seeds

Directions:

- ❖ Place all ingredients in a high speed blender and pulse until creamy.

Nutrition: Calories

Ingredients:

- ✓ ½ teaspoon ground cinnamon
- ✓ ¼ teaspoon ground ginger
- ✓ 1½ cups unsweetened almond milk
- ✓ ¼ cup ice cubes
- ❖ Pour the smoothie into two glasses and serve immediately.

81) Red fruit and vegetable smoothie

Preparation time: 10 minutes   **Cooking time**:   **Servings**: 2

Ingredients:

- ✓   ½ cup fresh raspberries
- ✓   ½ cup fresh strawberries
- ✓   ½ red bell pepper, seeded and chopped
- ✓   ½ cup red cabbage, chopped

Directions:

- ❖   Place all ingredients in a high speed blender and pulse until creamy.

Nutrition: Calories

Ingredients:

- ✓   1 small tomato
- ✓   1 cup of water
- ✓   ½ cup of ice cubes

- ❖   Pour the smoothie into two glasses and serve immediately.

82) Kale Smoothie

Preparation time: 10 minutes   **Cooking time**:   **Servings**: 2

Ingredients:

- ✓   3 fresh cabbage stalks, cut and chopped
- ✓   1-2 celery stalks, chopped
- ✓   ½ avocado, peeled, pitted and chopped

Directions:

- ❖   Place all ingredients in a high speed blender and pulse until creamy.

Nutrition: Calories

Ingredients:

- ✓   ½ inch ginger root, chopped
- ✓   ½ inch turmeric root, chopped
- ✓   2 cups of coconut milk

- ❖   Pour the smoothie into two glasses and serve immediately.

83) Green Tofu Smoothie

Preparation time: 10 minutes   **Cooking time**:   **Servings**: 2

Ingredients:

- ✓   1½ cups cucumber, peeled and coarsely chopped
- ✓   3 cups fresh spinach
- ✓   2 cups of frozen broccoli
- ✓   ½ cup silken tofu, drained and pressed

Directions:

- ❖   Place all ingredients in a high speed blender and pulse until creamy.

Nutrition: Calories

Ingredients:

- ✓   1 tablespoon fresh lime juice
- ✓   4-5 drops of liquid stevia
- ✓   1 cup unsweetened almond milk
- ✓   ½ cup ice, crushed
- ❖   Pour the smoothie into two glasses and serve immediately.

84) Grape and chard smoothie

Preparation time: 10 minutes   **Cooking time**:   **Servings**: 2

Ingredients:

- ✓   2 cups of green grapes without seeds
- ✓   2 cups fresh beets, cut and chopped
- ✓   2 tablespoons of maple syrup

Directions:

- ❖   Place all ingredients in a high speed blender and pulse until creamy.

Nutrition: Calories

Ingredients:

- ✓   1 teaspoon fresh lemon juice
- ✓   1½ cups of water
- ✓   4 ice cubes
- ❖   Pour the smoothie into two glasses and serve immediately.

85) Matcha Smoothie

Preparation time: 10 minutes   Cooking time: Servings: 2

Ingredients:

- ✓ 2 tablespoons of chia seeds
- ✓ 2 teaspoons of matcha green tea powder
- ✓ ½ teaspoon fresh lemon juice
- ✓ ½ teaspoon xanthan gum

Directions:

- ❖ Place all ingredients in a high speed blender and pulse until creamy.

Nutrition: Calories

Ingredients:

- ✓ 8-10 drops of liquid stevia
- ✓ 4 tablespoons of coconut cream
- ✓ 1½ cups unsweetened almond milk
- ✓ ¼ cup ice cubes
- ❖ Pour the smoothie into two glasses and serve immediately.

86) Banana Smoothie

Preparation time: 10 minutes   Cooking time: Servings: 2

Ingredients:

- ✓ 2 cups of cooled unsweetened almond milk
- ✓ 1 large frozen banana, peeled and sliced

Directions:

- ❖ Place all ingredients in a high speed blender and pulse until creamy.

Nutrition: Calories

Ingredients:

- ✓ 1 tablespoon almonds, chopped
- ✓ 1 teaspoon of organic vanilla extract
- ❖ Pour the smoothie into two glasses and serve immediately.

87) Strawberry Smoothie

Preparation time: 10 minutes   Cooking time: Servings: 2

Ingredients:

- ✓ 2 cups of cooled unsweetened almond milk
- ✓ 1½ cups of frozen strawberries

Directions:

- ❖ Add all ingredients to a high speed blender and pulse until smooth.

Nutrition: Calories

Ingredients:

- ✓ 1 banana, peeled and sliced
- ✓ ¼ teaspoon of organic vanilla extract
- ❖ Pour the smoothie into two glasses and serve immediately.

88) Raspberry and tofu smoothie

Preparation time: 15 minutes   Cooking time: Servings: 2

Ingredients:

- ✓ 1½ cups of fresh raspberries
- ✓ 6 ounces of firm silken tofu, drained
- ✓ 1/8 teaspoon of coconut extract

Directions:

- ❖ Add all ingredients to a high speed blender and pulse until smooth.

Nutrition: Calories

Ingredients:

- ✓ 1 teaspoon of stevia powder
- ✓ 1½ cups unsweetened almond milk
- ✓ ¼ cup ice cubes, crushed
- ❖ Pour the smoothie into two glasses and serve immediately.

89) Mango Smoothie

Preparation time: 10 minutes   Cooking time: Servings: 2

Ingredients:
- ✓ 2 cups frozen mango, peeled, pitted and chopped
- ✓ ¼ cup almond butter
- ✓ Pinch of ground turmeric

Ingredients:
- ✓ 2 tablespoons fresh lemon juice
- ✓ 1¼ cup unsweetened almond milk
- ✓ ¼ cup ice cubes
- ❖ Pour the smoothie into two glasses and serve immediately.

Directions:
- ❖ Add all ingredients to a high speed blender and pulse until smooth.

Nutrition: Calories

90) Pineapple Smoothie

Preparation time: 10 minutes   Cooking time: Servings: 2

Ingredients:
- ✓ 2 cups pineapple, chopped
- ✓ ½ teaspoon fresh ginger, peeled and chopped
- ✓ ½ teaspoon ground turmeric
- ✓ 1 teaspoon of natural immune support supplement*.

Ingredients:
- ✓ 1 teaspoon of chia seeds
- ✓ 1½ cups of cold green tea
- ✓ ½ cup ice, crushed
- ❖ Pour the smoothie into two glasses and serve immediately.

Directions:
- ❖ Add all ingredients to a high speed blender and pulse until smooth.

Nutrition: Calories

91) Cabbage and pineapple smoothie

Preparation time: 15 minutes   Cooking time: Servings: 2

Ingredients:
- ✓ 1½ cups fresh cabbage, chopped and shredded
- ✓ 1 frozen banana, peeled and chopped
- ✓ ½ cup of fresh pineapple chunks

Ingredients:
- ✓ 1 cup unsweetened coconut milk
- ✓ ½ cup of fresh orange juice
- ✓ ½ cup of ice
- ❖ Pour the smoothie into two glasses and serve immediately.

Directions:
- ❖ Add all ingredients to a high speed blender and pulse until smooth.

Nutrition: Calories

92) Green Vegetable Smoothie

Preparation time: 15 minutes   Cooking time: Servings: 2

Ingredients:
- ✓ 1 medium avocado, peeled, pitted and chopped
- ✓ 1 large cucumber, peeled and chopped
- ✓ 2 fresh tomatoes, chopped
- ✓ 1 small green bell pepper, seeded and chopped

Ingredients:
- ✓ 1 cup fresh spinach, torn
- ✓ 2 tablespoons fresh lime juice
- ✓ 2 tablespoons of homemade vegetable broth
- ✓ 1 cup of alkaline water
- ❖ Pour smoothie into glasses and serve immediately.

Directions:
- ❖ Add all ingredients to a high speed blender and pulse until smooth.

Nutrition: Calories

93) Avocado and spinach smoothie

Preparation time: 10 minutes   Cooking time: Servings: 2

Ingredients:

- ✓ 2 cups of fresh spinach
- ✓ ½ avocado, peeled, pitted and chopped
- ✓ 4-6 drops of liquid stevia

Directions:

- ❖ Add all ingredients to a high speed blender and pulse until smooth.

Nutrition: Calories

Ingredients:

- ✓ ½ teaspoon ground cinnamon
- ✓ 1 tablespoon of hemp seeds
- ✓ 2 cups of cooled alkaline water

- ❖ Pour the smoothie into two glasses and serve immediately.

94) Cucumber Smoothie

Preparation time: 15 minutes   Cooking time: Servings: 2

Ingredients:

- ✓ 1 small cucumber, peeled and chopped
- ✓ 2 cups fresh mixed greens (spinach, kale, chard), chopped and shredded
- ✓ ½ cup of lettuce, torn
- ✓ ¼ cup fresh parsley leaves
- ✓ ¼ cup fresh mint leaves

Directions:

- ❖ Add all ingredients to a high speed blender and pulse until smooth.

Nutrition: Calories

Ingredients:

- ✓ 2-3 drops of liquid stevia
- ✓ 1 teaspoon fresh lemon juice
- ✓ 1½ cups of filtered water
- ✓ ¼ cup ice cubes

- ❖ Pour the smoothie into two glasses and serve immediately.

95) Apple and Ginger Smoothie

Preparation time: 10 minutes   Cooking time: 0 minutes   Servings: 1

Ingredients:

- ✓ 1 apple, peeled and diced
- ✓ ¾ cup (6 ounces) of coconut yogurt

Directions:

- ❖ Add all ingredients to a blender.
- ❖ Blend well until smooth.

Nutrition: Calories

Ingredients:

- ✓ ½ teaspoon of ginger, freshly grated

- ❖ Refrigerate for 2 to 3 hours.
- ❖ Serve.

96) Green Tea Blueberry Smoothie

Preparation time: 10 minutes   Cooking time: 5 minutes   Servings: 1

Ingredients:

- ✓ 3 tablespoons of alkaline water
- ✓ 1 green tea bag
- ✓ 1 ½ cups fresh blueberries

Directions:

- ❖ Boil 3 tablespoons of water in a small saucepan and transfer to a cup.
- ❖ Dip the tea bag into the cup and let it sit for 4 to 5 minutes.
- ❖ Discard the tea bag and
- ❖ Transfer the green tea to a blender

Nutrition: Calories

Ingredients:

- ✓ 1 pear, peeled, stoned and diced
- ✓ ¾ cup of almond milk

- ❖ Add all other ingredients to blender.
- ❖ Blend well until smooth.
- ❖ Serve with fresh blueberries.

97) Apple and almond smoothie

Preparation time: 10 minutes

Cooking time: 0 minutes

Servings: 1

Ingredients:
- ✓ 1 cup of apple cider
- ✓ 1/2 cup of coconut yogurt
- ✓ 4 tablespoons almonds, crushed

Directions:
- ❖ Add all ingredients to a blender.

Nutrition: Calories

Ingredients:
- ✓ 1/4 teaspoon of cinnamon
- ✓ 1/4 teaspoon nutmeg
- ✓ 1 cup of ice cubes
- ❖ Blend well until smooth.
- ❖ Serve.

98) Cranberry Smoothie

Preparation time: 10 minutes

Cooking time: 0 minutes

Servings: 1

Ingredients:
- ✓ 1 cup of cranberries
- ✓ ¾ cup of almond milk
- ✓ ¼ cup raspberries

Directions:
- ❖ Add all ingredients to a blender.

Nutrition: Calories

Ingredients:
- ✓ 2 teaspoons fresh ginger, finely grated
- ✓ 2 teaspoons of fresh lemon juice

- ❖ Blend well until smooth.
- ❖ Serve with fresh berries on top.

99) Berry and Cinnamon Smoothie

Preparation time: 10 minutes

Cooking time: 0 minutes

Servings: 1

Ingredients:
- ✓ 1 cup of frozen strawberries
- ✓ 1 cup apple, peeled and diced
- ✓ 2 teaspoons fresh ginger
- ✓ 3 tablespoons of hemp seeds

Directions:
- ❖ Add all ingredients to a blender.

Nutrition: Calories

Ingredients:
- ✓ 1 cup of water
- ✓ ½ squeezed lime
- ✓ ¼ teaspoon of cinnamon powder
- ✓ ⅛ teaspoon of vanilla extract
- ❖ Blend well until smooth.
- ❖ Serve with fresh fruit

100) Detoxifying Berry Smoothie

Preparation time: 10 minutes

Cooking time: 0 minutes

Servings: 1

Ingredients:
- ✓ 3 peaches, with stone and peel
- ✓ 5 blueberries

Directions:
- ❖ Add all ingredients to a blender.

Nutrition: Calories

Ingredients:
- ✓ 5 raspberries
- ✓ 1 cup of alkaline water

- ❖ Blend well until smooth.
- ❖ Serve with fresh kiwi wedges.

Chapter 7 - Dr. Lewis's Meal Plan Project

Day 1

1) Mile Porridge

25) Zucchini salad

47) Carrot and celery soup

61) Cracker Healthy

33) Pasta salad with red lentils

Day 2

11) Cracker Pumpkin Spice

32) Cucumber salad

41) Potato and broccoli soup

68) Aquafaba

53) Zucchini, spinach and quinoa soup

Day 3

17) Cracker Healthy

39) Oatmeal, tofu and spinach burger

58) Spicy Eggplant

67) Walnut Milk homemade

31) Pad Thai Salad

Day 4

4) Squash Hash

22) Artichoke pie

55) Spinach Quinoa   2

77) Kiwi Smoothie

45) Pear and ginger soup

Day 5

6) Veggie Medley

27) Potato and pumpkin meatballs

45) Pear and ginger soup   2

79) Oatmeal and orange smoothie

29) Southern Salad

Day 6

6) Veggie Medley

39) Oatmeal, tofu and spinach burger

60) Cajun Zucchini seasoned   2

52) Zucchini and avocado soup with basil

21) Roasted artichoke salad

Day 7

13) Wheat Crackers

26) Fried tofu

50) Apple and sweet pumpkin soup

65) Blackberry Bars

36) Sweet potato salad with Jalapeno sauce

Chapter 8 -   Conclusion

I hope this book can lead you to your goals, keeping your desire to keep going high, without making you lose sight of the outcome

This book series is designed to help women, men, athletes and sportsmen, people immersed in work with little free time, etc.

If you recognize yourself in one of these categories or someone you know has decided to take the same path as you,

You'll find the other books in the series in your trusted bookstore, guaranteed!

Big hugs from Dr. Grace!